ALS: LOU GEHRIG'S DISEASE
PATIENT ADVOCATE

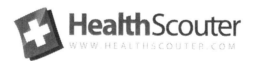

HealthScouter.com - Equity Press
5055 Canyon Crest Drive
Riverside, California 92507

www.healthscouter.com

Purchasing this book entitles you to free updates at
www.healthscouter.com/AmyotrophicLateralSclerosis

Edited By: Katrina Robinson

Includes Amyotrophic Lateral Sclerosis from Wikipedia
http://en.wikipedia.org/wiki/Amyotrophic_lateral_sclerosis

Important

NEVER DISREGARD PROFESSIONAL MEDICAL ADVICE, OR DELAY SEEKING IT, BECAUSE OF SOMETHING YOU HAVE READ IN THIS BOOK. ALWAYS SEEK PROFESSIONAL MEDICAL ADVICE BEFORE ACTING UPON INFORMATION READ IN THIS BOOK.

HealthScouter and Equity Press do not provide medical advice. The contents of this book are for informational purposes only and are not intended to substitute for professional medical advice, diagnosis or treatment. Always seek advice from a qualified physician or health care professional about any medical concern, and do not disregard professional medical advice because of anything you may read in this book or on a HealthScouter Web site. The views of individuals quoted in this book are not necessarily those of HealthScouter or Equity Press.

While this book is intended to be a medium for the exchange of information and ideas, it is not meant in any way to be a substitute for sound medical advice; neither should it be viewed as a trusted source of such advice. The views expressed in these messages are not those of any qualified medical association, and the publisher is not responsible for the validity of the information communicated herein or for consequences that may arise from acting upon this information. The publisher is not responsible for any content found in the book that may be deemed offensive, inappropriate, inaccurate or medically unsound. The information you find here is only for the purpose of discussion and should not be the basis for any medical decision. The content is not intended to be a substitute for professional medical advice, diagnosis or treatment.

The information presented is not to be considered complete, nor does it contain all medical resource information that may be relevant, and therefore it is not intended to be a substitute for seeking medical treatment and/or appropriate care.

By reading this book and parts of the Web site, you agree under all circumstances to hold harmless, and to refrain from seeking remedy from, the owners of this book. The publisher shall disclaim all liability to you for damages, costs or expenses, including legal and medical fees, related to your reliance on anything derived from this book or Web site or its contents. Furthermore, Equity Press assumes no liability for any and all claims arising out of the said use, regardless of the cause, effects, or fault.

Equity Press and HealthScouter do not endorse any company or product, and listing on the HealthScouter Web site is not linked to corporate sponsorship. We do not make a claim to being comprehensive or up to date. If you would like to recommend information to include in this book, please contact us – we would be very happy to hear from you.

Purchasing this book entitles you to free updates as they are available. Please register your book at www.healthscouter.com

TABLE OF CONTENTS

INTRODUCTION AND MOTIVATION

Dear Reader,

I like to think of myself as a polite, well-reasoned person. I rarely speak out or complain. When a waitress spills something on me, or if my meal is cold—or if I'm overcharged—I generally try to be as polite as possible. I don't like to make very many waves. I often secretly hope that the manager will hear about my predicament and come out and offer me a free meal, or something similar. I generally hope that my polite and respectful demeanor pays off. And it does happen from time to time. You know, I think many people are brought up to believe that this is just good manners. It's how you're supposed to behave. And if you knew me personally, I think you'd agree that I'm generally pretty reserved. Of course my wife may raise an objection or two (!), but I really believe that it's important to treat others as you would like to be treated. We're talking about the golden rule here—it works well and it applies to almost every life circumstance.

But I have to admit that when it comes to my health, or the health of someone I care about—all bets are off. I want to know what's going on—when, why, where, and how. And I make these feelings known. I tend to get downright assertive. It's just something I feel very strongly about. And I feel that when you are in a hospital, or if you're brushing up against the healthcare system, that you should feel the same way. It's unfamiliar turf, and the professionals who work in this system often take advantage of their positions. They may use some jargon to hide the whole truth— or they may say something without checking to make sure you understand completely. They may present the options that are best for them, perhaps the most profitable or convenient. Now I'm not saying this goes on everywhere. There are many professionals in the business of health who go out of their way to make sure you have the best care. And I'm not suggesting that you should become a bully, or purposefully annoying—absolutely not. But I am suggesting that I think it's OK for you to step outside of your typical comfort zone, and put on your patient advocate hat. Because you, the patient or patient advocate, care the most about your care—not the medical system or healthcare providers.

HealthScouter was created to help patients become better advocates for their own medical care. Because when it comes to your healthcare, the stakes are high. There are none higher. And healthcare is one area where consumers (us, the sick people) are notoriously unaware of their options. And that's why I'm publishing these books. To help you understand your options, and to help you get the best care possible. I want to help you become a better advocate for yourself and for your loved ones.

It's my sincere hope that you can take this book with you to the hospital, to be read in the waiting room or by the bedside—and when you see a relevant patient comment you can use this book to ask questions of your health care providers. My advice: Ask lots of questions! Providers are busy people who generally go about their business with little questioning, delivering care as they see fit—making quick decisions—and again, nobody is going to care as much about your health as you. So now, more than ever, you need tools at your disposal to get the best care possible. One of the tools at your disposal is this HealthScouter book and the material within. You need to be armed with questions, and you need to ask questions all of the time. And so the difficult part is now to understand the right questions to ask.

That brings me to an explanation of how these books are structured. HealthScouter books include a number of what we call patient comments. These patient comments are summaries of what people have experienced. They're first hand accounts of what you may expect. These experiences effectively help you "catch up," and understand what outcomes are possible. They expose you to the treatments are available, and provide insight as to potential outcomes. They help you understand what other people are doing. So if you find yourself stuck feeling like you're receiving substandard medical care—or if you need a push to broach the subject, you can take this book to your provider and say, "Hey, I read here that another patient had this treatment—is that an option for me? If not, Why?" I believe that other peoples' experience is the most valuable way for you to formulate and build a list of good questions for your healthcare providers.

That notion is at the core of the HealthScouter philosophy.

So HealthScouter, by providing patient comments about a particular medical condition, will help expose you to what other people have experienced about a particular medical problem. If you know what other people have experienced, you can better understand what your options are. You'll be better informed and you'll have some questions to ask—it'll be like you've had access to dozens of other people who have gone through the same thing you're going through. And so armed, maybe you'll be able to move through your condition and get back on the road to health, and maybe you'll be able to do this with more grace than I have. And that is my sincere wish.

It's also my wish that perhaps when a doctor or nurse sees this little blue book, that they'll think twice about the care they're about to provide—knowing that the owner is a little bit better prepared, a little bit better armed—and yes, maybe even downright assertive.

I hope this book helps.

Yours truly,

Jim Stewart

San Diego, California

HOW TO USE THIS BOOK

The purpose of HealthScouter is to help you understand your medical condition as quickly and easily as possible. We believe this can best be accomplished by reading about other people and their experiences negotiating their health and care. We try to leave out complicated medical jargon. And we've spent a considerable amount of time structuring this book so that it's easy to use. It's important to know that this is not the sort of book you read from beginning to end. Of course you may do so, but this book is more meaningful if you flip through quickly and scan for applicable material. Again, it's all about the patient commentary: The darkly shaded comments ▉ indicate one patient initiating a new discussion, and the light or clear comments ⬚ are other comments associated with that same condition. So you should begin by looking for information from other patients who are experiencing the same aspect of the same medical condition that you studying. You can do this quickly by scanning through the book, focusing on the dark shaded comment boxes. By scanning the patient comments you'll find information about various aspects of a condition, all grouped together, in an easy-to-read format. In this way you can immediately begin reading about other patients and their experiences with your particular medical condition – and you can benefit immediately from their experiences.

INTRODUCTION TO AMYOTROPHIC LATERAL SCLEROSIS

Amyotrophic lateral sclerosis (commonly referred to as ALS) is a form of motor neurone disease. Amyotrophic lateral sclerosis, sometimes called Maladie de Charcot, is a progressive,[1] fatal, neurodegenerative disease caused by the degeneration of motor neurons, the nerve cells in the central nervous system that control voluntary muscle movement. In the United States and Canada, the condition is often referred to as Lou Gehrig's Disease, after the New York Yankees baseball star who was diagnosed with the disease in 1939 and died from it in 1941, at age thirty-seven; today, renowned physicist Stephen Hawking is likely the best-known living amyotrophic lateral sclerosis patient. The disorder causes muscle weakness and atrophy throughout the body as both the upper and lower motor neurons degenerate, ceasing to send messages to muscles. Unable to function, the muscles gradually weaken, develop fasciculations (twitches) because of denervation, and eventually atrophy because of that denervation. The patient may ultimately lose the ability to initiate and control all voluntary movement; bladder and bowel sphincters and the muscles responsible for eye movement are usually (but not always) spared.

Cognitive function is generally spared except in certain situations such as when amyotrophic lateral sclerosis is associated with frontotemporal dementia.[2] However, there are reports of more subtle cognitive changes of the frontotemporal type in many patients when detailed neuropsychological testing is employed. Sensory nerves and the autonomic nervous system, which controls functions like sweating, generally remain functional.

I am a 39-year-old female. I have had a tendency toward fasciculations since childhood. In my early 20s I saw a neurologist who looked me over and pronounced them benign. I have always had them off and on but in the last month they have gone crazy. There isn't one moment all day where I cannot feel one in my leg, then stomach, then arm, back, neck, tongue, toe, hand, face. I have no weakness at all. I am very worried that I have amyotrophic lateral sclerosis. What does this sound like? Why the constant crazy fasciculations?

My neurologist told me that with amyotrophic lateral sclerosis, fasciculations are the last thing *that usually happens with the disease...that the muscles get weak first and the fasiculations happen FROM the muscles deteriorating after a while.*

Beginning a few months ago, I've gotten many strange symptoms that are scaring me to death.

- *Starting approximately one year ago, I've had a strange pain in my chest. It's a dull pain around the lower half of my left lung.*

- *My throat often gets sore*

- *Almost every major joint and muscle in my body gets very sore.*

- *My body has become very extremely snappy lately. Almost every joint makes a cracking noise at even the slightest movement.*

- *I feel drowsy often, and am unable to complete an entire day of work without becoming exhausted.*

- *Concentration problems.*

- *At times nausea, extreme tiredness.*

- *Recently the muscles in my face are tingling a bit.*

- *My tendons also feel tight all over my body.*

- *My heart races at times.*

Does this sound like amyotrophic lateral sclerosis to anyone?

No, it doesn't. It sounds more like lupus or fibromylagia. You might want to think about getting your thyroid checked. Low levels of thyroid hormone can cause a myriad of symptoms including extreme fatigue, muscle and joint aches and pains...basically a general feeling of being unwell.

SYMPTOMS

The initial onset of amyotrophic lateral sclerosis may be so subtle that the symptoms are frequently overlooked. The earliest symptoms are obvious weakness and/or muscle atrophy. This is followed by twitching, cramping, or stiffness of affected muscles; muscle weakness affecting an arm or a leg; and/or slurred and nasal speech. The twitching, cramping, etc. associated with amyotrophic lateral sclerosis is a result of the dying motor neurons, therefore these symptoms without clinical weakness or atrophy of affected muscle is likely not amyotrophic lateral sclerosis.

The parts of the body affected by early symptoms of amyotrophic lateral sclerosis depend on which motor neurons in the body are damaged first. About 75% of people experience "limb onset" amyotrophic lateral sclerosis. In some of these cases, symptoms initially affect one of the legs, and patients experience awkwardness when walking or running or they notice that they are tripping or stumbling more often. Other limb onset patients first see the effects of the disease on a hand or arm as they experience difficulty with simple tasks requiring manual dexterity such as buttoning a shirt, writing, or turning a key in a lock.

Occasionally the symptoms remain confined to one limb; this is known as monomelic amyotrophy.

About 25% of cases are "bulbar onset" amyotrophic lateral sclerosis. These patients first notice difficulty speaking clearly. Speech becomes garbled and slurred. Nasality and loss of volume are frequently the first symptoms. Difficulty swallowing, and loss of tongue mobility follow. Eventually total loss of speech and the inability to protect the airway when swallowing are experienced.

Regardless of the part of the body first affected by the disease, muscle weakness and atrophy spread to other parts of the body as the disease progresses. Patients experience increasing difficulty moving, swallowing (dysphagia), and speaking or forming words (dysarthria). Symptoms of upper motor neuron involvement include tight and stiff muscles (spasticity) and exaggerated reflexes (hyperreflexia) including an overactive gag reflex. An abnormal reflex commonly called Babinski's sign (the big toe extends upward and other toes spread out) also indicates upper motor neuron damage. Symptoms of lower motor neuron degeneration include muscle weakness and atrophy, muscle cramps, and fleeting twitches of muscles that can be seen under the skin (fasciculations). Around 15–45% of patients experience pseudobulbar affect, also known as "emotional lability", which consists of uncontrollable laughter, crying or smiling, attributable to degeneration of bulbar upper motor neurons resulting in exaggeration of motor expressions of emotion.

To be diagnosed with amyotrophic lateral sclerosis, patients must have signs and symptoms of both upper and lower motor neuron damage that cannot be attributed to other causes.

I am 24 and have some freaky symptoms I am scared about. I have muscle twitches everywhere! It moves my fingers sometimes. It is not localized. I noticed the first one four years ago, when I was writing a paper on amyotrophic lateral sclerosis. I also noticed some muscle loss, but that is hard to tell because I stopped working out. I am clumsy, but always was that. And now I am getting tingling in my feet. Should I be worried? Is amyotrophic lateral sclerosis connected to a positive ANA in blood work?

At your age and being female amyotrophic lateral sclerosis is unlikely. An MRI to rule out multiple sclerosis might be a good start.

I have been having some recent symptoms lately that slightly relate to the symptoms of amyotrophic lateral sclerosis. First, I have been having some weakness in my right hand, specifically in my index finger and thumb. Second, I have been having fasciculations in my left hand for about a month or so, in all of the fingers at this point. I noticed this week that my right hand is also having fasciculations now, only in the thumb. Does this sound like amyotrophic lateral sclerosis? What else can I look for?

Twitching is normally a sign that points away from amyotrophic lateral sclerosis. The mere fact that you are getting twitching in your left hand is a great sign. If you're noticing weakness in your right hand, the twitching would not occur in your left hand. The twitching, if you did have amyotrophic lateral sclerosis, would be one of the last things you would notice. The twitching in amyotrophic lateral sclerosis patients most times goes unnoticed. This is because the muscle tissue is dead, and they can not feel them.

You should get the hand checked out; chances are it is something simple.

I heard that amyotrophic lateral sclerosis symptoms are the same in ways as multiple sclerosis symptoms. Do you have numbness and other sensory feelings with amyotrophic lateral sclerosis?

I know somebody with amyotrophic lateral sclerosis and for the most part it doesn't seem to involve sensory neurons. He hasn't experienced any numbness or tingling-- progressive, irreversible muscle weakness only (due to neuron death). Most importantly, though, he has extreme muscle atrophy. I've heard it generally starts in one place, like the hand, and spreads from there.

I am a 25-year-old male. I started noticing twitches in my left arm two months ago but did not pay attention to it. The thing I am worried is that these twitches have become more precise. I can feel them and can even see them and now they are all over body. Now my legs are twitching and twitching in my arm has stopped.

Are these symptoms of amyotrophic lateral sclerosis?

I have been experiencing the same thing since May 2006. I went for two MRI scans, which were clear, and a visit to a neurologist; he said that there was nothing wrong with me.

A few months ago I stumbled upon Benign Fasciculation Syndrome while searching the internet for answers, and am convinced this is what I have. My symptoms started out with tingling in my hands and arms, and my legs felt like "jelly," as if they were going to give way. The muscle twitching started after that. I have read where people are experiencing the exact same symptoms as me and have Benign Fasciculation Syndrome.

Monomelic Amyotrophy

Monomelic amyotrophy (also known as MMA, Hirayama's disease, Sobue disease or Juvenile nonprogressive amyotrophy) is an untreatable, focal, lower motor neuron disease that primarily affects young (15–25-year-old) males in India and Japan. Monomelic amyotrophy is marked by insidious onset of muscular atrophy, which stabilizes at a plateau after two to five years from which it neither improves nor worsens. There is no pain or sensory loss associated with monomelic amyotrophy. Unlike other lower motor neuron diseases, monomelic amyotrophy is not believed to be hereditary and fasciculations (involuntary muscle twitches) are rare.

EMG tests reveal loss of the nerve supply, or denervation, in the affected limb without *conduction block* (nerve blockage restricted to a small segment of the nerve). Increased sweating, coldness and cyanosis have been reported for a few patients, indicating involvement of the sympathetic nervous system.

While monomelic amyotrophy will cause weakness and/or wasting in only one limb, EMG and NCV tests often show signs of reinnervation in the unaffected limbs.

I am a 40-year-old female who over the past several months developed sore wrists when I put weight on them. I also have muscle twitches all over my body for the past year. I went to my doctor and she did x-rays and blood work to look for arthritis. When this came back negative she sent me to a physiotherapist who noticed atrophy in both hands below my thumb. I have had one visit to the neurologist who agreed that I have focal atrophy in my hands, but did not find any weakness or any other signs of amyotrophic lateral sclerosis. He thinks it is likely related to carpal tunnel even though I don't have the typical wrist pain. He is sending me for an MRI, EMG/NCV and blood work and I see him in two months.

Has anyone ever heard of atrophy without severe weakness?

The EMG/NCS will tell whether you have carpal tunnel syndrome and would also reveal if you had ALS. I assume your neurologist ordered an MRI of your neck? Don't jump to any conclusions - you are on the young side to have amyotrophic lateral sclerosis, and this is a very rare condition.

I'm having some symptoms of amyotrophic lateral sclerosis and I'm hoping that someone can tell me other possible diseases that could cause these problems.

1. Approximately four weeks ago, I started to notice visible twitches...mainly on my left shoulder and right knee. In the last week or so, the twitches have not been as frequent, but they're still there.

2. Two weeks ago, I noticed my biceps and triceps felt weak in both arms, but much more so in my right arm. It really seemed to flare up during a stressful situation at work and never returned to normal. There is no visible atrophy and the weakness hasn't affected my daily life yet.

3. My legs, rib cage, and neck are sore on an off and on basis.

4. I have a tingling sensation on the back of my legs, my shins, my face, and my arms. It isn't constant, but enough to notice.

5. I'm not sure if this is related, but I've been running an on and off low-grade fever for the last month.

My regular doctor had me do physical tests and said he couldn't find anything wrong with me. He said it was probably an irritated nerve or a virus because of the fever. He said to call back in a few weeks if it isn't better so he could make arrangements with the clinic's neurologist.

I'm a 29-year-old man with no family history of diseases of this type. If anyone has any suggestions, I would be very thankful for your help.

You likely have what is called benign fasciculation syndrome, which is a form of peripheral nerve hyperexcitability. Although the cause is not specifically known, many patients exhibit elevate antibodies, suggesting an autoimmune origin. Muscle twitching in amyotrophic lateral sclerosis rarely preceeds significant weakness. When your *doctor performs a basic neurological exam, there are specific indicators of motor neuron disease that would be evident.*

Treatment

There is no cure for monomelic amyotrophy. Treatment consists of muscle strengthening exercises and training in hand coordination.

Prognosis

The symptoms of monomelic amyotrophy usually progress slowly for one to two years before reaching a plateau, and then remain stable for many years. Disability is generally slight. Rarely, the weakness progresses to the opposite limb. There is also a slowly progressive variant of monomelic amyotrophy known as O'Sullivan-McLeod syndrome, which only affects the small muscles of the hand and forearm and has a slowly progressive course.

Epidemiology

Monomelic amyotrophy occurs in males between the ages of 15 and 25. Onset and progression are slow. Monomelic amyotrophy is seen most frequently in Asia, particularly in Japan and India; it is much less common in North America.

Babinski's Sign

In medicine and neurology, the Babinski response to the plantar reflex is a reflex, named after Joseph Babinski (1857–1932), a French neurologist of Polish descent, that can identify disease of the spinal cord and brain and also exists as a primitive reflex in infants.[1][2] When non-pathological, it is called the plantar reflex, while the term Babinski's sign (or Koch's sign) refers to its pathological form.

Can anyone tell me about a positive Babinski's sign and what it may mean for me? My neurologist ordered an MRI test on my spine. I seem to trip all over myself all the time and indeed I'm getting scared.

According to my home medical encyclopedia, this is the entire description that is listed for it:

"A reflex movement in which the big toe bends upward when the outer edge of the sole of the foot is scratched. Babinski's sign indicates damage or disease of the brain or the spinal cord."

Since you are getting a spinal MRI, that must be where they believe there might be problems.

Methods

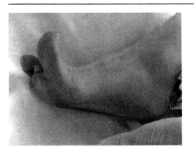

The above image shows a representation of Babinski's Sign

The lateral side of the sole of the foot is rubbed with a blunt instrument or device so as not to cause pain, discomfort or injury to the skin; the instrument is run from the heel along a curve to the toes[3] (metatarsal pads).

There are three responses possible:

• Flexor: the toes curve inward and the foot everts; this is the response seen in healthy adults (aka a "negative" Babinski)

• Indifferent: there is no response.

• Extensor: the hallux dorsiflexes and the other toes fan out - the "positive Babinski's sign" indicating damage to the central nervous system.

As the lesion responsible for the sign expands, so does the area from which the afferent Babinski response may be elicited. The Babinski response is also normal, while asleep and after a long period of walking.

 How many of you have a positive Babinski's reflex?

In people more than two years old, the presence of a Babinski's reflex indicates damage to the nerve paths connecting the spinal cord and the brain (the corticospinal tract). Because this tract is right-sided and left-sided, a Babinski's reflex can occur on one side or on both sides. I know that I had the reflex from 1982–1984 and have had it 24/7 since 2002.

The Babinski test is a standard Neurological tool used to measure reactions...the reaction is noted and checked each and every time that a neurological exam is performed.

Emerging symptoms

Although the sequence of emerging symptoms and the rate of disease progression vary from person to person, eventually patients will not be able to stand or walk, get in or out of bed on their own, or use their hands and arms. Difficulty swallowing and chewing impair the patient's ability to eat normally and increase the risk of choking. Maintaining weight will then become a problem. Because the disease usually does not affect cognitive abilities, patients are aware of their progressive loss of function and may become anxious and depressed. A small percentage of patients go on to develop frontotemporal dementia characterized by profound personality changes; this is more common among those with a family history of dementia. A larger proportion of patients experience mild problems with word-generation, attention, or decision-making. Cognitive function may be affected as part of the disease process or could be related to poor breathing at night (nocturnal hypoventilation). Health care professionals need to explain the course of the disease and describe available treatment options so that patients can make informed decisions in advance.

As the diaphragm and intercostal muscles (rib cage) weaken, forced vital capacity and inspiratory pressure diminish. In bulbar onset amyotrophic lateral sclerosis, this may occur before significant limb weakness is apparent. Bilevel positive pressure ventilation (frequently referred to by the tradename BiPAP) is frequently used to support breathing, first at night, and later during the daytime as well. It is recommended that long before bilevel positive pressure ventilation becomes insufficient, patients must decide whether to have a tracheostomy and long term mechanical ventilation. At this point, some patients choose palliative hospice care. Most people with amyotrophic lateral sclerosis die of respiratory failure or pneumonia, not the disease itself.

Amyotrophic lateral sclerosis predominantly affects the motor neurons, and in the majority of cases the disease does not impair a patient's mind, personality, intelligence, or memory. Nor does it affect a person's ability to see, smell, taste, hear, or feel touch. Control of eye muscles is the most preserved function, although some patients with an extremely long duration of disease (20+ years) may lose eye control too. Unlike multiple sclerosis, bladder and bowel control are usually preserved in amyotrophic lateral sclerosis, although as a result of immobility and diet changes, intestinal problems such as constipation can require intensive management.

I had slow speech problems for about three and a half months, but that went away after dumping a load of stressful items and anxieties on the floor to my parents and my wife about two weeks ago. I have been really worried about amyotrophic lateral sclerosis, but only being 33,

I think it is even rarer for it to be that. I had an EMG with very slight abnormalities with two muscles in my shoulder and one in my back, they tested approx 30 or more muscles. Shoulders rated a +1 and back rated a +2. My doctor said that this is extremely minor, but said that they could not rule out amyotrophic lateral sclerosis, due to my speech and the fasciculations which started during the EMG test. With my speech improving, I would like to hope that amyotrophic lateral sclerosis is being eliminated by the "lack of symptoms". Any suggestions?

Hang in there and keep a positive attitude. It's all in the attitude. I would suggest that you research Primary Lateral Sclerosis on the internet and ask your doctor about it.

I am a 42-year-old female. I have within the last year begun to have major muscle spasms and muscle twitches. They do not occur daily but when they do occur they will last any where from a couple days to a week or longer. They will occur in my calves, in both the front and back of my thighs, in my stomach, lower jaw and arms, and mainly in my right foot at the ball of my foot. My neck is always sore and at times feels like it takes a lot of effort to hold my head up. Any information will be most welcome.

It does sound like you have symptoms of amyotrophic lateral sclerosis, but it could also be something similar to it, some other kind of motor neuron problem. I would definitely go to a neurologist about it.

About two-three months ago, I was having twitches which lasted for almost a month; they came and went but then stopped completely. Then just recently I started having them again almost 24 hours a day for the last nine or ten days, almost always specifically in the same place in my upper right arm but rarely in other places as well. Recently the weakness came on very quickly. I noticed this weakness in my limbs all at the same time when I woke up in the morning the other day and it has not stopped. Will someone with ALS usually notice weakness in both the arms and legs at the same exact time, or does it usually start in one place and travel to another long after you first notice it?

Have you tested for Lyme's disease? I was diagnosed with amyotrophic lateral sclerosis and then found it was Lyme's. The two can easily be confused.

My husband was diagnosed with amyotrophic lateral sclerosis. His started in one limb and is slowly spreading to the other arm and leg. In the course of being diagnosed, we've found that several things can cause these symptoms such as stress, deficiencies, Lyme's disease, thyroid problems, infections, motor neuron disease, etc.

CAUSE AND RISK FACTORS

Scientists have not found a definitive cause for amyotrophic lateral sclerosis and the onset of the disease has been linked to several factors, including: a virus; exposure to neurotoxins or heavy metals; DNA defects; immune system abnormalities; and enzyme abnormalities. Surgeries involving the spinal cord have also been thought to play a role in the onset of amyotrophic lateral sclerosis due to the disruption of nerve fibers. There is a known hereditary factor in familial amyotrophic lateral sclerosis (FALS); however, there is no known hereditary component in the 90–95% cases diagnosed as sporadic amyotrophic lateral sclerosis. An inherited genetic defect on chromosome 21 is associated with approximately 20% of familial cases of amyotrophic lateral sclerosis.[3][4] This mutation is believed to be autosomal dominant. The children of those diagnosed with familial amyotrophic lateral sclerosis have a higher risk factor for developing the disease; however, those who have close family members diagnosed with sporadic amyotrophic lateral sclerosis have no greater a risk factor than the general population.[5]

Some causative factors have been suggested for the increased incidence in the western Pacific. Prolonged exposure to a dietary neurotoxin called BMAA is one suspected risk factor in Guam; the neurotoxin is a compound found in the seed of the cycad *Cycas circinalis*,[6] a tropical plant found in Guam, which was used in the human food supply during the 1950s and early 1960s.

The very high incidence of the disease among Italian soccer players (more than five times higher than normally expected) has raised the concern of a possible link between the disease and the use of pesticides on the soccer fields.[7][8]

According to the ALS Association, military veterans are at an increased risk of contracting amyotrophic lateral sclerosis. In its report *ALS in the Military*,[9] the group pointed to an almost 60% greater chance of the disease in military veterans than the general population. For Gulf War veterans, the chance is seen as twice that of veterans not deployed to the Persian Gulf in a joint study by the Veterans Affairs Administration and the DOD.[10][11]

Dietary intake of polyunsaturated fatty acids (PUFA) has been shown in several studies to decrease the risk of developing amyotrophic lateral sclerosis [12][13]

 I think amyotrophic lateral sclerosis is still a real possibility. My mom is 67. She had muscle weakness in her arms. Muscle fasciculation.

Loss of use of her left hand, now loss of use of her right. Her brain MRI showed some multiple sclerosis plaques; however, because of the muscle atrophy and fasciculation, the neurologist can't make a call between the two. He wants to conduct another MRI (because the emergency room doctor didn't use contrast). He also wants a more extensive EMG test. My mother is on cholesterol medication and triglyceride. I have just been reading about the dangers and possible linkage to these diseases. She was on Lipitor 20mg and was bumped to 40mg for a long time. She is now down to 20mg. Is there a confirmed linkage? Would stopping the meds even help at this point?

As far as I know it's never been proven that there's a link between statins and your mother's problems. Taking statins is pretty common, where as multiple sclerosis and amyotrophic lateral sclerosis are pretty uncommon diseases.

There are no studies recognized by the FDA that confirm a linkage; however, I have read many articles, written by doctors, that agree there could be a linkage because the statin drugs interfering with muscle cells, etc. There have also been studies that indicate statins are of no help for women or the elderly. They are most useful for middle aged men with heart disease. I don't know if stopping the statins would do any good at this time, but it couldn't hurt to start giving her CoQ10 supplement.

 My father is 47 and has amyotrophic lateral sclerosis. When I heard this from the doctor, I was really upset and crying. Will I get/inherit amyotrophic lateral sclerosis? My father is the only person in my family history that has this disease. Is the chance high?

It's not considered hereditary if there's only one person in your family that has it. A person's risk of getting amyotrophic lateral sclerosis is very low.

Only 10 percent of amyotrophic lateral sclerosis patients have a second family member who also has amyotrophic lateral sclerosis. Making it a 50 percent chance of a child getting amyotrophic lateral sclerosis. So the risk is lower with one person in a family like yourself. Chances are your dad is like the 90 percent who have an isolated family case of amyotrophic lateral sclerosis. Genetic testing can be done to determine if you have the gene.

PATHOPHYSIOLOGY

SOD1

The cause of amyotrophic lateral sclerosis is not known, though an important step toward answering that question came in 1993 when scientists discovered that mutations in the gene that produces the Cu/Zn superoxide dismutase (SOD1) enzyme were associated with some cases (approximately 20%) of familial amyotrophic lateral sclerosis. This enzyme is a powerful antioxidant that protects the body from damage caused by superoxide, a toxic free radical. Free radicals are highly reactive molecules produced by cells during normal metabolism. Free radicals can accumulate and cause damage to DNA and proteins within cells. Although it is not yet clear how the SOD1 gene mutation leads to motor neuron degeneration, researchers have theorized that an accumulation of free radicals may result from the faulty functioning of this gene. Current research, however, indicates that motor neuron death is not likely a result of lost or compromised dismutase activity, suggesting mutant SOD1 induces toxicity in some other way (a gain of function).[14][15]

Studies involving transgenic mice have yielded several theories about the role of SOD1 in mutant

SOD1 familial amyotrophic lateral sclerosis. Mice lacking the SOD1 gene entirely do not customarily develop amyotrophic lateral sclerosis, although they do exhibit an acceleration of age-related muscle atrophy (sarcopenia) and a shortened lifespan. This indicates that the toxic properties of the mutant SOD1 are a result of a gain in function rather than a loss of normal function. In addition, aggregation of proteins has been found to be a common pathological feature of both familial and sporadic amyotrophic lateral sclerosis. Interestingly, in mutant SOD1 mice, aggregates (misfolded protein accumulations) of mutant SOD1 were found only in diseased tissues, and greater amounts were detected during motor neuron degeneration.[16] It is speculated that aggregate accumulation of mutant SOD1 plays a role in disrupting cellular functions by damaging mitochondria, proteasomes, protein folding chaperones, or other proteins.[17] Any such disruption, if proven, would lend significant credibility to the theory that aggregates are involved in mutant SOD1 toxicity. Critics have noted that in humans, SOD1 mutations cause only 2% or so of overall cases and the etiological mechanisms may be distinct from those responsible for the sporadic form of the disease. To date, the amyotrophic lateral sclerosis-SOD1 mice remain the best model of the disease for preclinical studies but it hoped that more useful models will be developed.

Superoxide Dismutases

Superoxide dismutases (SOD, EC 1.15.1.1) are a class of enzymes that catalyze the dismutation of superoxide into oxygen and hydrogen peroxide. As such, they are an important antioxidant defense in nearly all cells exposed to oxygen. One of the exceedingly rare exceptions is *Lactobacillus plantarum* and related lactobacilli, which use a different mechanism.

Reaction

The SOD-catalysed dismutation of superoxide may be written with the following half-reactions :

- $M^{(n+1)+} - SOD + O_2^- \rightarrow M^{n+} - SOD + O_2$

- $M^{n+} - SOD + O_2^- + 2H^+ \rightarrow M^{(n+1)+} - SOD + H_2O_2.$

  where M = Cu (n=1) ; Mn (n=2) ; Fe (n=2) ; Ni (n=2).

In this reaction the oxidation state of the metal cation oscillates between n and n+1.

Biochemistry

Simply stated, SOD outcompetes damaging reactions of superoxide, thus protecting the cell from superoxide toxicity. The reaction of superoxide with non-radicals is spin forbidden. In biological systems, this means its main reactions are with itself (dismutation) or with another biological radical such as nitric oxide (NO). The superoxide anion radical (O_2^-) spontaneously dismutes to O_2 and hydrogen peroxide (H_2O_2) quite rapidly ($\sim 10^5$ M^{-1} s^{-1} at pH 7). SOD is biologically necessary because superoxide reacts even faster with certain targets such as NO radical, which makes peroxynitrite. Similarly, the dismutation rate is second order with respect to initial superoxide concentration. Thus, the half-life of superoxide, although very short at high concentrations (e.g. 0.05 seconds at 0.1mM) is actually quite long at low concentrations (e.g. 14 hours at 0.1 nM). In contrast, the reaction of superoxide with SOD is first order with respect to superoxide concentration. Moreover, superoxide dismutase has the fastest turnover number (reaction rate with its substrate) of any known enzyme ($\sim 7 \times 10^9$ M^{-1} s^{-1}),[6] this reaction being only limited by the frequency of collision between itself and superoxide. That is, the reaction rate is "diffusion limited".

Physiology

Superoxide is one of the main reactive oxygen species in the cell and as such, SOD serves a key antioxidant role. The physiological importance of SODs is illustrated by the severe pathologies evident in mice genetically engineered to lack these enzymes. Mice lacking SOD2 die several days after birth, amidst massive oxidative stress.[7] Mice lacking SOD1 develop a wide range of pathologies, including hepatocellular carcinoma,[8] an acceleration of age-related muscle mass loss,[9] an earlier incidence of cataracts and a reduced lifespan. Mice lacking SOD3 do not show any obvious defects and exhibit a normal lifespan, though they are more sensitive to hyperoxic injury.[10] Knockout mice of any SOD enzyme are more sensitive to the lethal effects of superoxide generating drugs, such as paraquat and diquat.

Drosophila lacking SOD1 have a dramatically shortened lifespan while flies lacking SOD2 die before birth. SOD knockdowns in C. elegans do not cause major physiological disruptions. Knockout or null mutations in SOD1 are highly detrimental to aerobic growth in the yeast Sacchormyces cerevisiae and result in a dramatic reduction in post-diauxic lifespan. SOD2 knockout or null mutations cause growth inhibition on respiratory carbon sources in addition to decreased post-diauxic lifespan.

Several prokaryotic SOD null mutants have been generated, including E. Coli. The loss of periplasmic

CuZnSOD causes loss of virulence and might be an attractive target for new antibiotics.

Other factors

Studies also have focused on the role of glutamate in motor neuron degeneration. Glutamate is one of the chemical messengers or neurotransmitters in the brain. Scientists have found that, compared to healthy people, amyotrophic lateral sclerosis patients have higher levels of glutamate in the serum and spinal fluid.[4] Laboratory studies have demonstrated that neurons begin to die off when they are exposed over long periods to excessive amounts of glutamate (excitotoxicity). Now, scientists are trying to understand what mechanisms lead to a buildup of unneeded glutamate in the spinal fluid and how this imbalance could contribute to the development of amyotrophic lateral sclerosis. Failure of astrocytes to sequester glutamate from the extracellular fluid surrounding the neurones has been proposed as a possible cause of this glutamate-mediated neurodegeneration.

Riluzole is currently the only FDA approved drug for amyotrophic lateral sclerosis and targets glutamate transporters. Its very modest benefit to patients has bolstered the argument that glutamate is not a primary cause of the disease. The antibiotic ceftriaxone has demonstrated an unexpected effect on glutamate and appears to be a beneficial treatment for amyotrophic lateral sclerosis in animal models. Ceftriaxone is currently being tested in clinical trials.

Autoimmune responses which occur when the body's immune system attacks normal cells have been suggested as one possible cause for motor neuron degeneration in amyotrophic lateral sclerosis. Some scientists theorize that antibodies may directly or indirectly impair the function of motor neurons, interfering with the transmission of signals between the brain and muscles. More recent evidence indicates that the nervous system's immune cells, microglia, are heavily involved in the later stages of the disease.

In searching for the cause of amyotrophic lateral sclerosis, researchers have also studied environmental factors such as exposure to toxic or infectious agents. Other research has examined the possible role of dietary deficiency or trauma. However, as of yet, there is insufficient evidence to implicate these factors as causes of amyotrophic lateral sclerosis.

Future research may show that many factors, including a genetic predisposition, are involved in the development of amyotrophic lateral sclerosis.

 I heard that Lyme disease can actually cause amyotrophic lateral sclerosis. Has anybody heard that or is that a rumor?

I have Lyme disease and have never heard this. Lyme disease is known as the great imitator because its symptoms mimic those of many other diseases including amyotrophic lateral sclerosis.

Diagnosis

No test can provide a definite diagnosis of amyotrophic lateral sclerosis, although the presence of upper and lower motor neuron signs in a single limb is strongly suggestive. Instead, the diagnosis of amyotrophic lateral sclerosis is primarily based on the symptoms and signs the physician observes in the patient and a series of tests to rule out other diseases. Physicians obtain the patient's full medical history and usually conduct a neurologic examination at regular intervals to assess whether symptoms such as muscle weakness, atrophy of muscles, hyperreflexia, and spasticity are getting progressively worse.

Because symptoms of amyotrophic lateral sclerosis can be similar to those of a wide variety of other, more treatable diseases or disorders, appropriate tests must be conducted to exclude the possibility of other conditions. One of these tests is electromyography (EMG), a special recording technique that detects electrical activity in muscles. Certain EMG findings can support the diagnosis of amyotrophic lateral sclerosis. Another common test measures nerve conduction velocity (NCV). Specific abnormalities in the NCV results may suggest, for example, that the patient has a form of peripheral neuropathy (damage to peripheral nerves) or myopathy (muscle disease) rather than amyotrophic lateral sclerosis. The physician may order magnetic resonance imaging (MRI), a noninvasive procedure that uses a magnetic field and radio waves to take detailed images of the brain and spinal cord. Although these MRI scans are often normal in patients with amyotrophic lateral sclerosis, they can reveal evidence of other problems that may be causing the symptoms, such as a spinal cord tumor, multiple sclerosis, a herniated disk in the neck, syringomyelia, or cervical spondylosis.

Based on the patient's symptoms and findings from the examination and from these tests, the physician may order tests on blood and urine samples to eliminate the possibility of other diseases as well as routine laboratory tests. In some cases, for example, if a physician suspects that the patient may have a myopathy rather than amyotrophic lateral sclerosis, a muscle biopsy may be performed.

Infectious diseases such as human immunodeficiency virus (HIV), human T-cell leukaemia virus (HTLV), Lyme disease,[18] syphilis[19] and tick-borne encephalitis[20] viruses can in some cases cause amyotrophic lateral sclerosis-like symptoms. Neurological disorders such as multiple sclerosis, , multifocal motor neuropathy, and spinal muscular atrophy also can mimic certain facets of the disease and should be considered by physicians attempting to make a diagnosis.

Because of the prognosis carried by this diagnosis and the variety of diseases or disorders that can resemble amyotrophic lateral sclerosis in the early stages of the disease, patients should always obtain a second neurological opinion.

A study by researchers from Mount Sinai School of Medicine identified three proteins that are found in significantly lower concentration in the cerebral spinal fluid of patients with amyotrophic lateral sclerosis than in healthy individuals. This finding was published in the February 2006 issue of Neurology. Evaluating the levels of these three proteins proved 95% accurate for diagnosing amyotrophic lateral sclerosis. The three protein markers are TTR, cystatin C, and the carboxyl-terminal fragment of neuroendocrine protein 7B2. These are the first biomarkers for this disease and may be first tools for confirming diagnosis of amyotrophic lateral sclerosis. With current methods, the average time from onset of symptoms to diagnosis is around 12 months. Improved diagnostic markers may provide a means of early diagnosis, allowing patients to receive relief from symptoms years earlier.[21]

I am a 30-year-old female. My symptoms started about three months ago. It started with my legs falling asleep while sitting. From what I read, pins and needles is not a symptom, but I would stand up and it would go away. Then it started while I was active, too, and then went into my arms! I would wake up with my limbs feeling like there was sand in them. My hands are very stiff, and I can't do simple things right like putting the cap on and off a razor, or cuting my food normally with a knife and fork. When I drive my car, my foot just does not want to apply pressure to the brake. An action normally not thought

about has actually become an effort. My hands
have worsened in the sense now when I hold
my pocketbook, which is heavy, my arms are
instantly tired and my hands/fingers shake. The
muscles in my legs are very sore, and I barely
have muscle but what is there is sore.

Two weeks ago another symptom started: muscle
twitching. At first it was not so much, but now it
is pretty much constant. I am normally a thin girl,
but I have lost more weight with no apparent
cause because I have not changed my eating
habits. I went from 105 to 95 in a few months,
and I look anorexic from the waist up. I am
now thinking the loss of weight is due to muscle
atrophy.

I went to a Neurologist who sent me for an MRI
on my brain (which came back normal), and
an MRI on cervical spine (normal except for
a herniated disc in my neck). Tomorrow I am
having the EMG. I understand this is the test that
would show amyotrophic lateral sclerosis, and I
feel I already know the answer. Are the results
instant? Will I know right away?

I believe you are going in the right direction to
discover your diagnosis. I think the EMG will be

one of the main test factors that will influence the diagnosis. Remember, amyotrophic lateral sclerosis symptoms are different for each individual, and may begin in different areas of the body; they might be severe for one person and less for the other.

My dad was told that there is a possibility that he has amyotrophic lateral sclerosis. All his test are good, but nerve conduction velocity test (NCV). Is it common for amyotrophic lateral sclerosis patients to show abnormalities in NCV test?

NCV are meant to be "normal" in amyotrophic lateral sclerosis, but if certain muscles are small (wasted) it will show as abnormal in amyotrophic lateral sclerosis.

My deceased grandfather was diagnosed with Landozy Degerine Muscular Dystrophy. I have now also. My concern is this...my symptoms are increasing quickly. The difficulty to swallow is increasing quickly and becoming quite irritating. My legs and arms are increasing in aching pain and my right ones have periodic twitches in which my husband advises my right arm twitches even more at night. I am 40 years old. I have a muscle biopsy upcoming. I have pulled my grandfather's medical records. He died at the age of 79 in 2000. In 1950 he was diagnosed by the Mayo clinic with amyotrophic lateral sclerosis. He would have been 29 yrs old. However, there is only ONE mention of it within his records. I am guessing it was an incorrect diagnosis. From my understanding and readings, death occurs within 3–5 yrs from diagnosis – is this right? I want to make sure that this is not a possibility of concern for me.

Never and I mean never have I heard of amyotrophic lateral sclerosis lasting 50 yrs. I think you are right it was a wrong diagnosis.

TREATMENT

No cure has yet been found.

I realize there are no medications available to cure amyotrophic lateral sclerosis. But are there medicines to slow progression? Medicines to regain any level of strength? Medicines to help with the fatigue? Is physically therapy helpful? Is diet helpful?

There is a treatment that has had good results in slowing the progression of amyotrophic lateral sclerosis, sometimes keeping its steady state. It's called "low dose naltrexone" or LDN. It is being used for a lot of autoimmune diseases including multiple sclerosis, fibromyalgia, Crohn's, cancer, etc. Not a wonder drug; it's the way it works on the immune system that allows it to help so many different problems. You have to find a sympathetic doctor who likes to try new things. No bad side effects, tiny dose of a drug that's usually given 50 mg, used at 3 - 4.5 mg. Also the medicine has to be compounded, not hard to do, just find the right pharmacy.

Medication

The Food and Drug Administration (FDA) has approved the first drug treatment for the disease: Riluzole (Rilutek). Riluzole is believed to reduce damage to motor neurons by decreasing the release of glutamate via activation of glutamate transporters. In addition, the drug offers a wide array of other neuroprotective effects, by means of sodium and calcium channel blockades,[22] inhibition of protein kinase C,[23] and the promotion of NMDA (N-methyl d-aspartate) receptor antagonism.[22][24] Clinical trials with amyotrophic lateral sclerosis patients showed that Riluzole lengthens survival by several months, and may have a greater survival benefit for those with a bulbar onset. The drug also extends the time before a patient needs ventilation support. Riluzole does not reverse the damage already done to motor neurons, and patients taking the drug must be monitored for liver damage and other possible side effects. However, this first disease-specific therapy offers hope that the progression of amyotrophic lateral sclerosis may one day be slowed by new medications or combinations of drugs. A small, open-label study recently suggested that the drug lithium which traditionally is used for the treatment of bipolar affective disorder may slow progression in both animal models and the human form of the disease.[25] However, further research is needed to establish whether the effect is real or not.

The tetracycline antibiotic minocycline is also under investigation for the treatment of amyotrophic lateral sclerosis among other neurological disorders. In rodents with the SOD1 gene mutation that has been associated with amyotrophic lateral sclerosis, Minocycline was as effective as Riluzole in extending survival, and it delayed the onset of movement problems.[26] It is thought to exert its neuroprotective effects not by affecting glutamate release as with Riluzole, but by inhibiting the release of a mitochondrial protein called cytochrome c into the body of the cell.

The new discovery of RNAi has some promise in treating amyotrophic lateral sclerosis. In recent studies, RNAi has been used in lab rats to shut off specific genes that lead to amyotrophic lateral sclerosis. Cytrx Corporation has sponsored amyotrophic lateral sclerosis research utilizing RNAi gene silencing technology targeted at the mutant SOD1 gene.[27] The mutant SOD1 gene is responsible for causing amyotrophic lateral sclerosis in a subset of the 10% of all amyotrophic lateral sclerosis patients who suffer from the familial, or genetic, form of the disease. Cytrx's orally-administered drug Arimoclomol is currently in clinical evaluation as a therapeutic treatment for amyotrophic lateral sclerosis.

Insulin-like growth factor 1 has also been studied as treatment for amyotrophic lateral sclerosis. Cephalon and Chiron conducted two pivotal clinical studies of IGF-1 for amyotrophic lateral sclerosis, and although one study demonstrated efficacy, the second was equivocal, and the product has never been approved by the FDA. In January 2007, the Italian Ministry of Health has requested INSMED corporation's drug, IPLEX, which is a recombinant IGF-1 with Binding Protein 3(IGF1BP3) to be used in a clinical trial for amyotrophic lateral sclerosis patients in Italy.

Methylcobalamin is being studied in Japan;[28] preliminary results show it significantly lengthens survival time of amyotrophic lateral sclerosis patients.

A close relative was just diagnosed with amyotrophic lateral sclerosis and is given less than a few short years to live. The medication will only extend life for about ninety days. I have read some testimonials from people who claim to have overcome it by changing their diet or gaining spirituality or detoxifying their bodies. Is there any truth to this or does anyone know of anything that might help?

You might look into Low Dose Naltrexone. I've been taking it for the last four years myself to help curtail the progression of my multiple sclerosis.

Riluzole

Riluzole is a drug used to treat amyotrophic lateral sclerosis. It delays the onset of ventilator-dependence or tracheostomy in selected patients and may increase survival by approximately three to five months.

It is marketed by sanofi-aventis with the brand name Rilutek.

Mechanism of action

Riluzole has several actions:

• Sodium channel blockade

• High-voltage calcium channel blockade

• N-methyl-D-aspartate (NMDA)/glutamate receptor antagonism

• Glutamate transporter activation

• Inhibition of protein kinase C

Riluzole preferentially blocks TTX sensitive sodium channels, which are associated with damaged neurons.[1] This reduces influx of calcium ions and indirectly prevents stimulation of glutamate receptors. Together with direct glutamate receptor blockade, the effect of the neurotransmitter glutamate on motor neurons is greatly reduced.

However, the action of riluzole on glutamate receptors has been controversial, as no binding of the molecule has been shown on any known receptor.[2] In addition as its antiglutamate action is still detectable in the presence of sodium channel blockers, it is also uncertain whether or not it acts via this way. Rather, its potent glutamate uptake activator activity seems to mediate many of its effects.[3][4]

 Is anyone taking Rilutek? My mom was diagnosed in April and we think she might have Lyme disease on top of amyotrophic lateral sclerosis. They prescribed her Rilutek, but she's yet to take it. What are the pros and cons?

I was diagnosed with amyotrophic lateral sclerosis in 2002. I told my doctors that I had an imbedded tick in 2000. Neither one of them listened to me and tested for Lyme! I was offered the rilutex and refused to take it because of the side effects (liver

damage). My advice is to go to a Lyme expert only.

Studies of efficacy

A Cochrane Library review states a 9% gain in the probability of surviving one year. In secondary analyses of survival at separate time points, there was a significant survival advantage with riluzole 100 mg at six, nine, 12 and 15 months, but not at three or 18 months.[5] There was a small beneficial effect on both bulbar and limb function, but not on muscle strength. There were no data on quality of life, but patients treated with riluzole remained in a more moderately affected health state significantly longer than placebo-treated patients.

Clinical use

While riluzole has been proven to slow down amyotrophic lateral sclerosis, patients do not report any subjective improvement. Approximately 10% of patients experience side effects such as nausea and fatigue which lead them to discontinue treatment. Safety monitoring includes regular liver function tests and people with liver disease such as hepatitis should be monitored especially carefully.

In the UK riluzole has been available through the NHS since 1997 at a standard dosage of 50 mg twice daily. There has been some evidence to show that higher doses might produce more significant improvements in amyotrophic lateral sclerosis patients but at £5 a tablet it is at risk of being prohibitively expensive given the modest benefit to patients. One study in the Netherlands found that riluzole is metabolised differently by males and females, and its levels in plasma are decreased in patients who smoke cigarettes.[6]

A number of recent case studies have also indicated that riluzole may have clinical use in mood and anxiety disorders. It has been shown to have antidepressant properties in the treatment of refractory depression[7] and as an anxiolytic in Obsessive-compulsive disorder[8] and in GAD

Arimoclomol

Arimoclomol (INN, originally codenamed BRX-220) is an experimental drug developed by CytRx Corporation, a biopharmaceutical company based in Los Angeles, California. The orally administered drug is intended to treat amyotrophic lateral sclerosis.[1][2]

Mechanism of action

Arimoclomol is believed to function by stimulating a normal cellular protein repair pathway through the activation of molecular chaperones. Since damaged proteins, called aggregates, are thought to play a role in many diseases, CytRx believes that arimoclomol could treat a broad range of diseases.

Arimoclomol activates the heat shock response.[3][4][5][6][7][8] It is believed to act at Hsp70.[9]

History

Arimoclomol has been shown to extend life in an animal model of amyotrophic lateral sclerosis[10] and was well tolerated in healthy human volunteers in a Phase I study. CytRx is currently conducting a Phase II clinical trial.[11]

Arimoclomol was discovered by Hungarian researchers, as a drug candidate to treat insulin resistance[12][13] and diabetic complications such as retinopathy, neuropathy and nephropathy. Later, the compound, along with other small molecules, was screened for further development by Hungarian firm Biorex, which was sold to CytRx Corporation, who developed it toward a different direction from 2003.

IPLEX

IPLEX (mecasermin rinfabate [rDNA origin] injection) is a drug consisting of synthetic Insulin-like growth factor 1 (IGF-1) and insulin-like growth factor binding protein-3 (IGFBP-3).[1][2]

It is believed to be similar in effect to mecasermin, but with fewer side effects (such as hypoglycemia)

Potential uses

It was developed by INSMED corporation for the treatment of growth failure in children with severe primary IGF-I deficiency (Primary IGFD) or with growth hormone (GH) gene deletion who have developed neutralizing antibodies to GH. Due to a patent settlement, IPLEX is being taken off the market for short stature related indications. However, IPLEX is being studied as a treatment for other several serious medical conditions.

On March 11, 2009 the FDA announced that mecaserim would be made available to Americans with amyotrophic lateral sclerosis, more commonly known as Lou Gehrig's disease, as a part of a clinical trial. The drug is currently available in Italy for this condition.[4][5]

In January 2007, INSMED announced that the Italian Ministry of Health requested INSMED corporation to make IPLEX available to treat Italian patients sufferings from amyotrophic lateral sclerosis.

However IGF-1, the main component of IPLEX was the subject of a recent clinical trial in amyotrophic lateral sclerosis. It involved 330 people with amyotrophic lateral sclerosis from 20 amyotrophic lateral sclerosis treatment centres across the United States. The drug was injected under the skin (subcutaneous delivery) in a randomized double-blinded placebo-controlled trial – this is the gold standard way of conducting a clinical trial. At the end of the two-year treatment period, there were no differences between people with amyotrophic lateral sclerosis who received IGF-1 and those who received placebo in muscle strength, the need for a tracheostomy for breathing, or survival, indicating that IGF-1 provided patients no benefit. The current results are published in the November 25 issue of Neurology.[6] The researchers were led by Eric J. Sorenson, MD, from the Mayo Clinic in Rochester, Minnesota *"While this is very disappointing, at least it was definitive and gives, I think, a pretty definitive answer, at least for this strategy for this drug,"* Dr. Sorenson said.[7] However, he added, *"there is still a great deal of evidence that the IGF-1 pathway can be beneficial to people who have amyotrophic lateral sclerosis, but just not the way we administered it."*

Novel methods of delivering IGF-1 in a more selected fashion are now under way, including the use of viral mediators or stem cells. Two previous phase 3 trials of IGF-1 in amyotrophic lateral sclerosis showed inconsistent results: 1 trial, carried out in North America, did find a benefit, whereas the other, a European trial, did not confirm the earlier findings. "The results of our study most resemble those of the previous European study, with no benefit in either survival or functional scales,", De Sorenson concludes. "It is disappointing that we were unable to confirm the benefit that was noted in the previous North American study."

Methylcobalamin

Methylcobalamin is a cobalamin (MeB_{12}) used in peripheral neuropathy, diabetic neuropathy etc. It is a form of vitamin B_{12}. This vitamer is one of two active coenzymes used by B-12 dependent enzymes in the body, and is specifically the B-12 form used by 5-methyltetrahydrofolate-homocysteine methyltransferase (MTR), also known as methionine synthase.

Methylcobalamin has been studied in conjunction with sleep-wake rhythm disorders, where it appears to yield benefits, but at a low or inconsistent level.[1]

It is used in treating diseases of vitamin B12 deficiency (such as pernicious anemia), or diseases of effective B12 deficiency, such as vitamin B12 metabolic pathway pathologies.

One study suggests that once absorbed, methylcobalamin may be retained in the body better than cyanocobalamin.

Other

Other treatments for amyotrophic lateral sclerosis are designed to relieve symptoms and improve the quality of life for patients. This supportive care is best provided by multidisciplinary teams of health care professionals such as physicians; pharmacists; physical, occupational, and speech therapists; nutritionists; social workers; and home care and hospice nurses. Working with patients and caregivers, these teams can design an individualized plan of medical and physical therapy and provide special equipment aimed at keeping patients as mobile and comfortable as possible.

Physicians can prescribe medications to help reduce fatigue, ease muscle cramps, control spasticity, and reduce excess saliva and phlegm. Drugs also are available to help patients with pain, depression, sleep disturbances, and constipation. Pharmacists can advise on best use of medications. This is particularly helpful with regards to patients with dysphagia, which many amyotrophic lateral sclerosis patients experience. They would also monitor a patient's medications to reduce risk of drug interactions.

Physical therapy and special equipment such as assistive technology can enhance patients' independence and safety throughout the course of amyotrophic lateral sclerosis. Gentle, low-impact aerobic exercise such as walking, swimming, and stationary bicycling can strengthen unaffected muscles, improve cardiovascular health, and help patients fight fatigue and depression. Range of motion and stretching exercises can help prevent painful spasticity and shortening (contracture) of muscles. Physical therapists can recommend exercises that provide these benefits without overworking muscles.

Physiotherapists can suggest devices such as ramps, braces, walkers, and wheelchairs that help patients remain mobile. Occupational therapists can provide or recomment equipment and adaptations to enable people to retain as much independence in activities of daily living as possible.

Amyotrophic lateral sclerosis patients who have difficulty speaking may benefit from working with a speech-language pathologist. These health professionals can teach patients adaptive strategies such as techniques to help them speak louder and more clearly. As amyotrophic lateral sclerosis progresses, speech-language pathologists can recommend the use of augmentative and alternative communication such as voice amplifiers, speech-generating devices (or voice output communication devices) and/or low tech communication techniques such as alphabet boards or yes/no signals. These methods and devices help patients communicate when they can no longer speak or produce vocal sounds. With the help of occupational Therapists, speech-generating devices can be activated by switches or mouse emulation techniques controlled by small physical movements of, for example, the head, finger or eyes.

Patients and caregivers can learn from speech-language pathologists and nutritionists how to plan and prepare numerous small meals throughout the day that provide enough calories, fiber, and fluid and how to avoid foods that are difficult to swallow.

Patients may begin using suction devices to remove excess fluids or saliva and prevent choking. When patients can no longer get enough nourishment from eating, doctors may advise inserting a feeding tube into the stomach. The use of a feeding tube also reduces the risk of choking and pneumonia that can result from inhaling liquids into the lungs. The tube is not painful and does not prevent patients from eating food orally if they wish.

When the muscles that assist in breathing weaken, use of nocturnal ventilatory assistance (intermittent positive pressure ventilation (IPPV) or bilevel positive airway pressure (BIPAP)) may be used to aid breathing during sleep. Such devices artificially inflate the patient's lungs from various external sources that are applied directly to the face or body. When muscles are no longer able to maintain oxygen and carbon dioxide levels, these devices may be used full-time.

Patients may eventually consider forms of mechanical ventilation (respirators) in which a machine inflates and deflates the lungs. To be effective, this may require a tube that passes from the nose or mouth to the windpipe (trachea) and for long-term use, an operation such as a tracheostomy, in which a plastic breathing tube is inserted directly in the patient's windpipe through an opening in the neck. Patients and their families should consider several factors when deciding whether and when to use one of these options. Ventilation devices differ in their effect on the patient's quality of life and in cost. Although ventilation support can ease problems with breathing and prolong survival, it does not affect the progression of amyotrophic lateral sclerosis. Patients need to be fully informed about these considerations and the long-term effects of life without movement before they make decisions about ventilation support. It must be pointed out that some patients under long-term tracheostomy intermittent positive pressure ventilation with deflated cuffs or cuffless tracheostomy tubes (leak ventilation) are able to speak. This technique preserves speech in some patients with long-term mechanical ventilation.

Social workers and home care and hospice nurses help patients, families, and caregivers with the medical, emotional, and financial challenges of coping with amyotrophic lateral sclerosis, particularly during the final stages of the disease. Social workers provide support such as assistance in obtaining financial aid, arranging durable power of attorney, preparing a living will, and finding support groups for patients and caregivers. Home nurses are available not only to provide medical care but also to teach caregivers about tasks such as maintaining respirators, giving feedings, and moving patients to avoid painful skin problems and contractures. Home hospice nurses work in consultation with physicians to ensure proper medication, pain control, and other care affecting the quality of life of patients who wish to remain at home. The home hospice team can also counsel patients and caregivers about end-of-life issues.

Both animal and human research suggest calorie restriction (CR) may be contraindicated for those with amyotrophic lateral sclerosis. Research on a transgenic mouse model of amyotrophic lateral sclerosis demonstrates that calorie restriction may hasten the onset of death in amyotrophic lateral sclerosis.[29] In that study, Hamadeh *et al.* also note two human studies[30][31] that they indicate show "low energy intake correlates with death in people with amyotrophic lateral sclerosis." However, in the first study, Slowie, Paige, and Antel state: "The reduction in energy intake by amyotrophic lateral sclerosis patients did not correlate with the proximity of death but rather was a consistent aspect of the illness." They go on to conclude: "We conclude that amyotrophic lateral sclerosis patients have a chronically deficient intake of energy and recommended augmentation of energy intake."[30]

Previously, Pedersen and Mattson also found that in the amyotrophic lateral sclerosis mouse model, calorie restriction "accelerates the clinical course" of the disease and had no benefits.[32] Suggesting that a calorically dense diet may slow amyotrophic lateral sclerosis, a ketogenic diet in the amyotrophic lateral sclerosis mouse model has been shown to slow the progress of disease.[33]

Will a person with amyotrophic lateral sclerosis lose the ability to move their eyes? What can I expect from amyotrophic lateral sclerosis?

My father had amyotrophic lateral sclerosis and was diagnosed when I was 11 years old. I remember he first began to need a cane when walking and was given only five years. His speech began to slur after about a year and only immediate family could understand him. After two years he started losing muscles in his hands and was not able to drive. He then began to lose his speech more and more and was writing like a preschooler. The best thing to do is have someone learn how to understand them and be able to translate so they don't get frustrated when trying to speak or communicate. One of the best pieces of advice I can give you is that my father began eating only natural foods and using holistic treatments and herbal remedies and he stayed alive for an extra three years.

He did begin to get glaucoma and was 95% blind in one eye and 5% in the other but it wasn't until year five or so this happened. He eventually also lost ability to swallow and needed tubes.

 I lost my father and youngest brother to amyotrophic lateral sclerosis a year apart. Is there anyone out there who had similar losses? I am looking for a support group in my area but no luck yet.

Do you want to meet face to face with other people? Have you contacted your local hospital? Often they have knowledge of support groups from which you might be able to benefit.

How exactly does amyotrophic lateral sclerosis kill you?

Amyotrophic lateral sclerosis is the muscle wasting and hardening of voluntary muscles. You can hold your breath, cough, and swallow voluntarily; eventually these muscles will be effected. It is my understanding that a person with amyotrophic lateral sclerosis will likely die from respritory complications.

A person with amyotrophic lateral sclerosis usually succumbs to carbon dioxide poisoning. This is a bi-product that we normally breathe out during exhalation. A person with amyotrophic lateral sclerosis eventually gets where the lungs and breathing is too weak to put off this product and this eventually causes respiratory failure. Use of a BiPap does help to prolong the build up of the CO_2 (Carbon dioxide), but eventually the lungs do shut completely down.

Under some circumstances a person with amyotrophic lateral sclerosis can succumb to choking or pneumonia- however they usually pass away from the CO_2 build-up/respiratory failure.

PROGNOSIS

Regardless of the part of the body first affected by the disease, it is usual for muscle weakness and atrophy to spread to other parts of the body as the disease progresses. It is important to remember that some patients with amyotrophic lateral sclerosis have an arrested course with no progression beyond a certain point despite extensive follow-up. Such a pattern is particularly true for young males with predominant upper limb weakness especially on one side (so-called monomelic or Hirayama type motor neuron disease). Eventually people with amyotrophic lateral sclerosis will not be able to stand or walk, get in or out of bed on their own, or use their hands and arms. In later stages of the disease, individuals have difficulty breathing as the muscles of the respiratory system weaken. Although ventilation support can ease problems with breathing and prolong survival, it does not affect the progression of amyotrophic lateral sclerosis. Most people with amyotrophic lateral sclerosis die from respiratory failure, usually within 3–5 years from the onset of symptoms. However, about 10 percent of those individuals with amyotrophic lateral sclerosis survive for 10 or more years.

Does anyone know how what the life expectancy is for someone diagnosed with amyotrophic lateral sclerosis and who has started to decline in health?

The life expectancy is 2–5 years.

Please seek professional advice. Some lose use of limbs first and then the voice, others just the reverse. Everyone is different and timeframes are also different. Generally for most of us life expectancy as a rule is 2–5 years after diagnosis.

What are the signs that the patient is in the last stage of amyotrophic lateral sclerosis?

This is very hard to say with amyotrophic lateral sclerosis. I have had several friends die and they had high FVC's. Most are going to die when they have respiratory failure.

EPIDEMIOLOGY

Amyotrophic lateral sclerosis is one of the most common neuromuscular diseases worldwide, and people of all races and ethnic backgrounds are affected. One to two people per 100,000 develop amyotrophic lateral sclerosis each year.[34] Amyotrophic lateral sclerosis most commonly strikes people between 40 and 60 years of age, but younger and older people can also develop the disease. Men are affected slightly more often than women.

"Familial amyotrophic lateral sclerosis" accounts for approximately 5%–10% of all amyotrophic lateral sclerosis cases and is caused by genetic factors. Of these, approximately 1 in 10 are linked to a mutation in copper/zinc superoxide dismutase (SOD1), an enzyme responsible for scavenging free radicals. A recent study has identified a gene called FUS ("Fused in Sarcoma", ALS6) as being responsible for 1 in 20 cases of familial amyotrophic lateral sclerosis.[35][36]

Although the incidence of amyotrophic lateral sclerosis is thought to be regionally uniform, there are three regions in the West Pacific where there has in the past been an elevated occurrence of amyotrophic lateral sclerosis. This seems to be declining in recent decades. The largest is the area of Guam inhabited by the Chamorro people, who have historically had a high incidence (as much as 143 cases per 100,000 people per year) of a condition called Lytico-Bodig disease which is a combination of amyotrophic lateral sclerosis, Parkinsonism, and dementia.[37] Two more areas of increased incidence are the Kii peninsula of Japan and West Papua.[38][39]

Although there have been reports of several "clusters" including three American football players from the San Francisco 49ers, more than fifty soccer players in Italy [40], three soccer-playing friends in the south of England,[41] and reports of conjugal (husband and wife) cases in the south of France,[42][43][44][45][46] these are statistically plausible chance events. Although many authors consider amyotrophic lateral sclerosis to be caused by a combination of genetic and environmental risk factors, so far the latter have not been firmly identified, other than a higher risk with increasing age.

I'm 15 years old. My muscles have been twitching for the past week. My arms feel numb. I have shortness of breath. Do my symptoms sound like amyotrophic lateral sclerosis?

It would be VERY unusual for somebody your age to get amyotrophic lateral sclerosis. You should go and see a doctor, but it sounds like you are having an anxiety attack at the moment. There is a condition called benign fasciculation, which means muscle-twitching. You may have that. Go and get the symptoms checked out to make you feel better.

There are other conditions that mimic amyotrophic lateral sclerosis; fibromyalgia and Lyme's disease are but two of these conditions. I would encourage you to see a doctor to rule out obvious problems... supplement your magnesium because low levels don't show up on the tests that doctors use (and deficiencies cause some of the symptoms you describe).

ETYMOLOGY

Amyotrophic comes from the Greek language: A-means "no", *myo* refers to "muscle", and *trophic* means "nourishment"; *amyotrophic* therefore means "no muscle nourishment," which describes the characteristic atrophication of the sufferer's disused muscle tissue. *Lateral* identifies the areas in a person's spinal cord where portions of the nerve cells that are affected are located. As this area degenerates it leads to scarring or hardening ("sclerosis") in the region.

HISTORY

Timeline	
Year	Event
1850	English scientist Augustus Waller describes the appearance of shriveled nerve fibers
1869	French doctor Jean-Martin Charcot first describes amyotrophic lateral sclerosis in scientific literature
1881	"On Amyotrophic Lateral Sclerosis" is translated into English and published in a three-volume edition of Lectures on the Diseases of the Nervous System
1939	Amyotrophic lateral sclerosis becomes a *cause célèbre* in the United States when baseball legend Lou Gehrig's career — and, two years later, his life — are ended by the disease.
1950s	Amyotrophic lateral sclerosis epidemic occurs among the Chamorro people on Guam
1991	Researchers link chromosome 21 to familial amyotrophic lateral sclerosis
1993	SOD1 gene on chromosome 21 found to play a role in some cases of familial amyotrophic lateral sclerosis
1996	Rilutek becomes the first FDA-approved drug for amyotrophic lateral sclerosis
1998	El Escorial is developed as the standard for confirming amyotrophic lateral sclerosis
2001	Alsin gene on chromosome 2 found to cause ALS2

MOTOR NEURON DISEASE

The motor neurone diseases (or motor neuron diseases) (MND) are a group of neurological disorders that selecively affect motor neurones,[1] the cells that control voluntary muscle activity including speaking, walking, breathing, swallowing and general movement of the body.

> *Can anyone please tell me what Motor Neuron Syndrome is? I am guessing and hoping it is not the same as Motor Neuron Disease.*
>
> *I am currently have tests to determine what is wrong with me but have been sent a letter saying I have Motor Neuron Syndrome and further tests should identify the cause.*

> *It's nonspecific. Means you have signs and symptoms that suggest a problem with your motor neurons. You won't know any more until you have those tests.*

Terminology

In this article, motor neuron disease refers to a group of diseases that affect motor neurones. In the United States, *motor neuron disease* is more commonly called *Amyotrophic lateral sclerosis*, or *Lou Gehrig's disease*, after the baseball player.[1] In France the disease is sometimes known as *Maladie de Charcot* (Charcot's disease), although it may also be referred to by the direct translation of amyotrophic lateral sclerosis, Sclerose Laterale Amyotrophique (SLA). To avoid confusion, the annual scientific research conference dedicated to the study of motor neuron disease is called the International ALS/MND Symposium.

Classification

Forms of motor neurone disease include:

• amyotrophic lateral sclerosis

• primary lateral sclerosis (PLS)

• progressive muscular atrophy (PMA)

• bulbar[2]

  • pseudobulbar palsy - spastic

  • progressive bulbar palsy - spastic and flaccid

Spinal muscular atrophy (SMA) is classified under motor neuron disease by MeSH, but not by ICD-10.

Complications

Labile Affect

Labile affect or pseudobulbar affect refers to the pathological expression of laughter, crying, or smiling. It is also known as emotional lability, pathological laughter and crying, emotional incontinence, or, more recently, involuntary emotional expression disorder (IEED).[1] Patients may find themselves laughing uncontrollably at something that is only moderately humorous, being unable to stop themselves for several minutes. Episodes may also be mood-incongruent: a patient might laugh uncontrollably when angry or frustrated, for example.

Labile affect is most commonly observed after brain injury, people with dementia expressing a psychosis of some sort, or degeneration in amyotrophic lateral sclerosis (also known as Lou Gehrig disease), a form of motor neuron disease. It affects up to 50% of patients or up to 17,000 people, particularly those with pseudobulbar palsy.[2] It also occurs in approximately 10% of multiple sclerosis patients[3], signalling a degree of cognitive impairment. It is also currently being considered for inclusion in the DSM as one of the two symptoms (of five possible) which must be present for a diagnosis of ADHD in adults.

While not as profoundly disabling as the physical symptoms of these diseases, labile affect can have a significant impact on individuals' social functioning and their relationships with others. In motor neuron disease, the majority of patients are cognitively normal; however, the appearance of uncontrollable emotions is commonly associated with learning disabilities. This may lead to severe embarrassment and avoidance of social interactions for the patient, which in turn has an impact on their coping mechanisms and their careers.

Treatment for labile affect is usually pharmacological, using antidepressants such as fluoxetine, citalopram, or amitriptyline in low to moderate doses. In the USA, a combination of dextromethorphan and a subtherapeutic dose of quinidine has been submitted to the U.S. Food and Drug Administration (FDA) for approval to treat emotional lability.

Extra-motor change

Cognitive change occurs in between 33–50% of patients. A small proportion exhibit a form of frontotemporal dementia characterised by behavioural abnormalities such as disinhibition, apathy, and personality changes. A small proportion of patients may also suffer from an aphasia, which causes difficulty in naming specific objects. A larger proportion (up to 50%) suffer from a milder version of cognitive change which primarily affects what is known as executive function. Briefly, this is the ability of an individual to initiate, inhibit, sustain, and switch attention and is involved in the organisation of complex tasks down to smaller components. Often patients with such changes find themselves unable to do the family finances or drive a car. Depression is surprisingly rare in motor neuron disease (around 5–20%) relative to the frequency with which it is found in other, less severe, neurological disorders e.g. ~50% in multiple sclerosis and Parkinson's disease, ~20% in Epilepsy. Depression does not necessarily increase as the symptoms progress, and in fact many patients report being happy with their quality of life despite profound disability. This may reflect the use of coping strategies such as reevaluating what is important in life.

Although traditionally thought only to affect the motor system, sensory abnormalities are not necessarily absent, with some patients finding altered sensation to touch and heat, found in around 10% of patients. Patients with a predominantly upper motor neurone syndrome, and particularly PLS, often report an enhanced startle reflex to loud noises.

Neuroimaging and neuropathology has demonstrated extra-motor changes in the frontal lobes including the inferior frontal gyrus, superior frontal gyrus, anterior cingulate cortex, and superior temporal gyrus. The degree of pathology in these areas has been directly related to the degree of cognitive change experienced by the patient, if any. Patients with motor neuron disease and dementia have been shown to exhibit marked frontotemporal lobe atrophy as revealed by MRI or SPECT neuroimaging.

I'm a 25-year-old female. My symptoms started about four weeks ago. I noticed a slight weak feeling in my thighs and biceps. Several days later I had 27/7 vertigo, which I think has something to do with my inner ear. I've had several bouts of vertigo on and off for the past three years. The vertigo has lessoned, but the weakness seems to be getting worse. I also notice that when I'm typing or writing my hands tire much quicker as if I've been typing or writing for hours.

My physician did some blood work everything came back normal except for an increase in my ALT levels (liver related). She told me if symptoms persist, she will order an MRI.

Do any of these things sound like amyotrophic lateral sclerosis?

Have your doctor order the MRI now. Tell her you're worried, your symptoms aren't better and that it would put your mind at ease to get it done sooner than later. They usually will do it if it is reasonable and you're firm but nice.

As far as ALS symptoms, weakness, muscle fasiculations, and clumsiness are a few of the first signs from what I've read. There are several types of amyotrophic lateral sclerosis. The fastest progressing is bulbar type; that usually starts with your throat, swallowing, etc.

There are many things that can cause your symptoms. Multiple sclerosis, amyotrophic lateral sclerosis, stress, deficiencies, Lyme's disease, and infections are just a few.

ALS ASSOCIATION

The ALS Association is an American non profit organization that raises money for research and patient services, promotes awareness about and advocates in state and federal government on issues related to amyotrophic lateral sclerosis. The ALS Association is broken up into distinct chapters each servicing a particular geographic area of the United States all working under the umbrella of a national charter and administrator. While each individual chapter is basically autonomous, some smaller chapters rely heavily on the national organization for assistance. Each chapter provides education, advocacy and essential services to amyotrophic lateral sclerosis patients, their families and caregivers, while the national organization funds research and supports the cause as a whole.

Mission

The stated mission of The ALS Association is "To lead the fight to cure and treat ALS through global, cutting edge research, and to empower people with Lou Gehrig's Disease and their families to live fuller lives by providing them with compassionate care and support."

Vision & Values

In the quest to create a world without amyotrophic lateral sclerosis, the vision of The ALS Association is to "care for and support all people living with Lou Gehrig's Disease and leave no stone unturned in a relentless search for a cure."

The ALS Association says that they will achieve their vision by upholding a commitment to be the:

- Preeminent organization and catalyst in directing, funding and promoting amyotrophic lateral sclerosis research.

- Most comprehensive provider of care and support services to the amyotrophic lateral sclerosis Community through our coordinated network of Chapters, Centers and clinics.

- Leading advocate and voice for the amyotrophic lateral sclerosis Community.

- Recognized authority and most trusted source of information and education about amyotrophic lateral sclerosis.

The values of The ALS Association are as follows:

- People with amyotrophic lateral sclerosis and their families come first in everything we do.

- Scientific credibility and innovation are the hallmarks of our research program.

- Integrity, honesty and ethical behavior guide all our endeavors.

- Champion the cause of people with amyotrophic lateral sclerosis to raise awareness, understanding and support at every turn.

- Collaboration and partnership within our organization and with others who share our goals and values promote continued success in the fight against amyotrophic lateral sclerosis.

- Mutual respect is the cornerstone for all our working relationships.

- Financial strength enables us to accomplish our goals.

- Commitment to excellence and professionalism are key tenets at all levels of our organization.

- Diversity of ideas, cultures, ethnicities and backgrounds strengthen our efforts.

- Teamwork: We are a unified organization with one vision and one mission.[1]

Research

The ALS Association drives amyotrophic lateral sclerosis research through:

- Funding international research programs from basic to clinical research

- The organization of scientific workshops to stimulate scientific collaborations and bring new scientists to the amyotrophic lateral sclerosis field and

- Rapid translation of findings into clinical trials for amyotrophic lateral sclerosis patients.

Twice annually, The ALS Association invites researchers to submit proposals for consideration. The Association awards multi-year and starter grants as well as an annual post-doctoral fellowship. At any given time there are approximately 100 Association-funded research studies in progress. The ALS Association also initiates scientific studies through its ALS Association-initiated research program. Launched in 2000, this effort complements and works in tandem with the investigator-initiated research by engaging established investigators with extensive expertise and applying the most advanced technology to answer the more complex questions about amyotrophic lateral sclerosis.

TREAT ALS Program

The ALS Association's TREAT ALS (Translational Research Advancing Therapy for Amyotrophic Lateral Sclerosis)[2] initiative combines efficient new drug discovery with priorities set for existing drug candidates, to accelerate clinical testing of compounds with promise for the disease. Already partnering with many organizations around the world including The National Institutes of Health (NIH), The ALS Association brings together an expert team of scientific and business advisors to steer this import drug discovery program.

Amyotrophic Lateral Sclerosis Research Workshops

Amyotrophic lateral sclerosis focused workshops for the scientific community are hosted by The ALS Association during the year to advance current knowledge about the mechanisms and cause(s) of amyotrophic lateral sclerosis, attract more neuroscientists to amyotrophic lateral sclerosis research and foster collaborative research.

The ALS Association Certified Center Program

The mission of The ALS Association Center[SM] Program is to define, establish and support a national standard of care in the management of amyotrophic lateral sclerosis, sponsored by The ALS Association.
The objective of the ALS Center Program is to encourage and provide state-of-the-art care and clinical management of amyotrophic lateral sclerosis through:

• The involvement of all necessary healthcare disciplines in the care of the amyotrophic lateral sclerosis patient and family

• The offering of care from a team of people specially trained to meet the needs of those living with amyotrophic lateral sclerosis, regardless of the ability to pay; and

• Collaborative work among Centers to enhance amyotrophic lateral sclerosis patient care and techniques

The ALS Association selects, certifies and supports distinguished regional institutions recognized as the best in the field with regard to knowledge of and experience with amyotrophic lateral sclerosis; and which have neurological diagnostics and imaging, and available on-site licensed and certified ancillary services on clinic days including (but not limited to):

- Physical therapy

- Occupational therapy

- Respiratory therapy

- Nursing

- Registered dietician services

- Ph.D. psychology or psychiatry

- Speech and language pathology

- Social Work

Advocacy

The ALS Association network plays a lead role in advocacy for increased public and private support of amyotrophic lateral sclerosis research and health care reform that responds to the demands imposed by amyotrophic lateral sclerosis.

Advocacy for research, health & long-term care, and caregiver support is the primary function of the Advocacy Department of The ALS Association. Based in Washington, D.C., The ALS Association's Capital Office coordinates the federal and state advocacy program, works directly with Congress, the White House, other federal agencies and other national organizations, and provides training and support for ALS Association advocates.

The Capital Office also organizes The ALS Association's National Advocacy Day and Public Policy Conference each year. This event is the amyotrophic lateral sclerosis community's only opportunity to join together to educate Members of Congress on the importance of stepping up the fight to conquer amyotrophic lateral sclerosis through research, care and support.

Every May during ALS Awareness Month, the ALS Association leads a contingent of amyotrophic lateral sclerosis patients, advocates, and caregivers to Capitol Hill for a National ALS Advocacy Day and Public Policy Conference. In 2007, more than 800 people visited Washington, D.C. from 39 states, to raise awareness of amyotrophic lateral sclerosis.

The ALS Association's advocacy efforts in Washington, D.C. have raised the profile of amyotrophic lateral sclerosis at the White House, among members of Congress, and within federal agencies, including the National Institutes of Health, the Food and Drug Administration, and the Social Security

Administration. Participation of advocates throughout the amyotrophic lateral sclerosis community resulted in amyotrophic lateral sclerosis being included with only twenty-eight other diseases in the Department of Defense 2003 Appropriations bill $50 million Peer Reviewed Medical Research Program.

In an historic victory for the amyotrophic lateral sclerosis community, their efforts led Congress to waive the 24-month waiting period for Medicare coverage of people diagnosed with amyotrophic lateral sclerosis as part of the fiscal year 2001 spending bill. Elimination of this waiting period will positively affect the lives of people with amyotrophic lateral sclerosis and provide them access to the care they need in a timely manner.

Other victories include:

• Passage of The ALS Registry Law that established the first national registry in which doctors can report new cases of amyotrophic lateral sclerosis (ALS).[3]

• Making amyotrophic lateral sclerosis a presumptive illness in the VA that allows veterans who contract amyotrophic lateral sclerosis compensation through the government. The VA also provides compensation to surviving spouses of Veterans who died from amyotrophic lateral sclerosis.[4]

Chapters

The ALS Association chapter is a multi-faceted grass-roots organization that carries out The ALS Association's mission and strategic goals at the community level.[5] The chapter - with supporting services from the National Office - actively pursues The Association's goals by providing a wide range of services for people living with amyotrophic lateral sclerosis, their caregivers, families and friends as well as professional health care providers throughout the service area. Each ALS Association chapter offers programs that can include many of the following:

- Patient education programs

- Support groups

- Telephone information/referral service

- Equipment loan programs

- Augmentative communication device programs

- Respite programs

- Programs of information and support for caregivers and family members

- Referrals to amyotrophic lateral sclerosis clinics and physicians

- Support nationally-directed research programs

- Local and nationally-directed advocacy programs

Walk to Defeat Amyotrophic Lateral Sclerosis

The Walk to Defeat Amyotrophic Lateral Sclerosis is The ALS Association's national signature event. Each year, over 100,000 people including amyotrophic lateral sclerosis patients, families, friends and corporate leaders join together to raise funds in support of The Association's cutting-edge research and community-based patient services programs. Approximately 150 walks will be held around the country in 2008.[6]

REFERENCES – AMYOTROPHIC LATERAL SCLEROSIS

1. *amyotrophic lateral sclerosis* at Dorland's Medical Dictionary

2. Phukan J, Pender NP, Hardiman O (2007). "Cognitive impairment in amyotrophic lateral sclerosis". *Lancet Neurol* **6** (11): 994–1003. doi:10.1016/ S1474-4422(07)70265-X. PMID 17945153. http://linkinghub.elsevier.com/ retrieve/pii/S1474-4422(07)70265-X.

3. Conwit, Robin A. (December 2006). "Preventing familial ALS: A clinical trial may be feasible but is an efficacy trial warranted?". *Journal of the Neurological Sciences* **251** (1–2): 1–2. doi:10.1016/j.jns.2006.07.009. ISSN 0022-510X.

4. Al-Chalabi, Ammar; P. Nigel Leigh (August 2000). "Recent advances in amyotrophic lateral sclerosis". *Current Opinion in Neurology* **13** (4): 397–405. ISSN 1473-6551. PMID 10970056.

5. http://web.archive.org/web/20041115214832/http://www.alsphiladelphia. org/pennstatehershey/newsletters/newsletter_spring04.htm

6. Khabazian I, Bains JS, Williams DE, Cheung J, Wilson JM, Pasqualotto BA, Pelech SL, Andersen RJ, Wang YT, Liu L, Nagai A, Kim SU, Craig UK, Shaw CA (August 2002). "Isolation of various forms of sterol beta-D-glucoside from the seed of Cycas circinalis: neurotoxicity and implications for ALS-parkinsonism dementia complex". *J. Neurochem.* **82** (3): 516–28. PMID 12153476. http:// www3.interscience.wiley.com/resolve/openurl?genre=article&sid=nlm: pubmed&issn=0022-3042&date=2002&volume=82&issue=3&spage=516. Retrieved on 2009-03-13.

7. "Sla, indagini nei club. Pesticidi nel mirino". http://www.corriere.it/sport/08_ ottobre_03/sla_indagine_pesticidi_fd04f986-911c-11dd-9f28-00144f02aabc. shtml. Retrieved on 2008-10-02.

8. "Sla, una strage nel calcio". http://www.gazzetta.it/Calcio/Altro_Calcio/ Primo_Piano/2007/11_Novembre/30/sla_3011.shtml. Retrieved on 2008-10-02.

9. "ALS in the Military". The ALS Association. 2007-05-17. http://www.alsa.org/ files/pdf/als_military_paper.pdf. Retrieved on 2008-05-01.

10. "Occurrence of ALS higher in Gulf War veterans". http://www.bcm.edu/ fromthelab/vol02/is10/03oct_n1.htm.

11. "Veterans get ALS disability". http://www.baltimoresun.com/news/nation/ bal-te.als25jul25,0,7448073.story.

12. Veldink JH, Kalmijn S, Groeneveld GJ, Wunderink W, Koster A, de Vries JH, van der Luyt J, Wokke JH, Van den Berg LH (April 2007). "Intake of polyunsaturated fatty acids and vitamin E reduces the risk of developing amyotrophic lateral sclerosis". *J. Neurol. Neurosurg. Psychiatr.* **78** (4): 367–71. doi:10.1136/ jnnp.2005.083378. PMID 16648143. http://jnnp.bmj.com/cgi/pmidlookup?view =long&pmid=16648143. Retrieved on 2009-03-13.

13. Okamoto K, Kihira T, Kondo T, Kobashi G, Washio M, Sasaki S, Yokoyama T, Miyake Y, Sakamoto N, Inaba Y, Nagai M (October 2007). "Nutritional status and risk of amyotrophic lateral sclerosis in Japan". *Amyotroph Lateral Scler* **8** (5): 300–4. doi:10.1080/17482960701472249. PMID 17852010. http://www.informaworld.com/openurl?genre=article&doi=10.1080/17482960701472249&magic=pubmed‖1B69BA326FFE69C3F0A8F227DF8201D0. Retrieved on 2009-03-13.

14. Reaume A, Elliott J, Hoffman E, Kowall N, Ferrante R, Siwek D, Wilcox H, Flood D, Beal M, Brown R, Scott R, Snider W (1996). "Motor neurons in Cu/Zn superoxide dismutase-deficient mice develop normally but exhibit enhanced cell death after axonal injury". *Nat Genet* **13** (1): 43–7. doi:10.1038/ng0596-43. PMID 8673102.

15. Bruijn L, Houseweart M, Kato S, Anderson K, Anderson S, Ohama E, Reaume A, Scott R, Cleveland D (1998). "Aggregation and motor neuron toxicity of an ALS-linked SOD1 mutant independent from wild-type SOD1". *Science* **281** (5384): 1851–4. doi:10.1126/science.281.5384.1851. PMID 9743498.

16. Furukawa Y, Fu R, Deng H, Siddique T, O'Halloran T (2006). "Disulfide cross-linked protein represents a significant fraction of ALS-associated Cu, Zn-superoxide dismutase aggregates in spinal cords of model mice". *Proc Natl Acad Sci U S a* **103** (18): 7148–53. doi:10.1073/pnas.0602048103. PMID 16636274.

17. Boillée S, Vande Velde C, Cleveland D (2006). "ALS: a disease of motor neurons and their nonneuronal neighbors". *Neuron* **52** (1): 39–59. doi:10.1016/j.neuron.2006.09.018. PMID 17015226.

18. Hansel Y, Ackerl M, Stanek G. (1995). "ALS-like sequelae in chronic neuroborreliosis". *Wien Med Wochenschr.* **145** (7-8): 186–8. PMID 7610670.

19. el Alaoui-Faris M, Medejel A, al Zemmouri K, Yahyaoui M, Chkili T (1990). "Amyotrophic lateral sclerosis syndrome of syphilitic origin. 5 cases". *Rev Neurol (Paris)* **146** (1): 41–4. PMID 2408129.

20. Umanekii KG, Dekonenko EP (1983). "Structure of progressive forms of tick-borne encephalitis". *Zh Nevropatol Psikhiatr Im S S Korsakova.* **83** (8): 1173–9. PMID 6414202.

21. Pasinetti G, Ungar L, Lange D, Yemul S, Deng H, Yuan X, Brown R, Cudkowicz M, Newhall K, Peskind E, Marcus S, Ho L (2006). "Identification of potential CSF biomarkers in ALS". *Neurology* **66** (8): 1218–22. doi:10.1212/01.wnl.0000203129.82104.07. PMID 16481598.

22. Hubert JP, Delumeau JC, Glowinski J, Prémont J, Doble A. (1994). "Antagonism by riluzole of entry of calcium evoked by NMDA and veratridine in rate cultured granule cells: evidence for a dual mechanism of action". *Br. J. Pharmacol.* **113** (1): 261–267. PMID 7812619.

23. Noh KM, Hwang JY, Shin HC, Koh JY. (2000). "A Novel Neuroprotective Mechanism of Riluzole: Direct Inhibition of Protein Kinase C". *Neurobiol Dis.* **7** (4): 375–383. doi:10.1006/nbdi.2000.0297. PMID 10964608.

24. Beal MF, Lang AE, Ludolph AC. (2005). *Neurodegenerative Diseases: Neurobiology, Pathogenesis and Therapeutics.* Cambridge: Cambridge University Press. p. p. 775. ISBN 0-521-81166-X. OCLC 57691713.

25. Fornai F, Longone P, Cafaro L, *et al.* (2008). "Lithium delays progression of amyotrophic lateral sclerosis". *Proc. Natl. Acad. Sci. U.S.A.* **105**: 2052. doi:10.1073/pnas.0708022105. PMID 18250315. http://www.pnas.org/cgi/pmidl ookup?view=long&pmid=18250315.

26. [1]

27. Xia X, Zhou H, Huang Y, Xu Z (Sep 2006). "Allele-specific RNAi selectively silences mutant SOD1 and achieves significant therapeutic benefit in vivo". *Neurobiol Dis.* **23** (3): 578–86. doi:10.1016/j.nbd.2006.04.019. PMID 16857362.

28. Izumi Y, Kaji R (October 2007). "[Clinical trials of ultra-high-dose methylcobalamin in ALS]" (in Japanese). *Brain Nerve* **59** (10): 1141–7. PMID 17969354.

29. Hamadeh MJ, Rodriguez MC, Kaczor JJ, Tarnopolsky MA (Feb 2005). "Caloric restriction transiently improves motor performance but hastens clinical onset of disease in the Cu/Zn-superoxide dismutase mutant G93A mouse". *Muscle Nerve* **31** (2): 214–20. doi:10.1002/mus.20255. PMID 15625688.

30. Kasarskis EJ, Berryman S, Vanderleest JG, Schneider AR, McClain CJ (Jan 1996). "Nutritional status of patients with amyotrophic lateral sclerosis: relation to the proximity of death". Am J Clin Nutr. **63** (1): 130–7. PMID 8604660. http://www.ajcn.org/cgi/pmidlookup?view=long&pmid=8604660.

31. Slowie LA, Paige MS, Antel JP (Jul 1983). "Nutritional considerations in the management of patients with amyotrophic lateral sclerosis (ALS)". *J Am Diet Assoc* **83** (1): 44–7. PMID 6863783.

32. Pedersen WA, Mattson MP (Jun 1999). "No benefit of dietary restriction on disease onset or progression in amyotrophic lateral sclerosis Cu/Zn-superoxide dismutase mutant mice". *Brain Res.* **833** (1): 117–20. doi:10.1016/S0006-8993(99)01471-7. PMID 10375685. http://linkinghub.elsevier.com/retrieve/pii/S0006-8993(99)01471-7.

33. Zhao Z, Lange DJ, Voustianiouk A, *et al.* (2006). "A ketogenic diet as a potential novel therapeutic intervention in amyotrophic lateral sclerosis". *BMC Neurosci* **7**: 29. doi:10.1186/1471-2202-7-29. PMID 16584562. Media report on Zhao *et al.*.

34. "ALS Topic Overview". http://www.webmd.com/brain/tc/Amyotrophic-Lateral-Sclerosis-ALS-Topic-Overview. Retrieved on 2008-05-01.

35. Vance C, Rogelj B, Hortobágyi T, De Vos KJ, Nishimura AL, Sreedharan J, Hu X, Smith B, Ruddy D, Wright P, Ganesalingam J, Williams KL, Tripathi V, Al-Saraj S, Al-Chalabi A, Leigh PN, Blair IP, Nicholson G, de Belleroche J, Gallo JM, Miller CC, Shaw CE (February 2009). "Mutations in FUS, an RNA processing protein, cause familial amyotrophic lateral sclerosis type 6". *Science (journal)* **323** (5918): 1208–11. doi:10.1126/science.1165942. PMID 19251628. http://www. sciencemag.org/cgi/pmidlookup?view=long&pmid=19251628. Retrieved on 2009-03-13.

36. Kwiatkowski TJ, Bosco DA, LeClerc AL, Tamrazian E, Vanderburg CR, Russ C, Davis A, Gilchrist J, Kasarskis EJ, Munsat T, Valdmanis P, Rouleau GA, Hosler BA, Cortelli P, de Jong PJ, Yoshinaga Y, Haines JL, Pericak-Vance MA, Yan J, Ticozzi N, Siddique T, McKenna-Yasek D, Sapp PC, Horvitz HR, Landers JE, Brown, RH (Feb 2009). "Mutations in the FUS/TLS Gene on Chromosome 16 Cause Familial Amyotrophic Lateral Sclerosis". *Science* **323** (5918): 1205-1208. doi:10.1126/science.1166066.

37. Reed D, Labarthe D, Chen KM, Stallones R (Jan 1987). "A cohort study of amyotrophic lateral sclerosis and parkinsonism-dementia on Guam and Rota". *Am J Epidemiol.* **125** (1): 92–100. PMID 3788958. http://aje. oxfordjournals.org/cgi/pmidlookup?view=long&pmid=3788958.

38. S. Kuzuhara, Y. Kokubo P3-146Marked increase of parkinsonism-dementia (P-D) phenotypes in the high incidence amyotrophic lateral sclerosis (ALS) focus in the Kii peninsula of Japan. Alzheimer's and Dementia, Volume 2, Issue 3, Pages S417-S417

39. Spencer PS, Palmer VS, Ludolph AC (Aug 2005). "On the decline and etiology of high-incidence motor system disease in West Papua (southwest New Guinea)". *Mov. Disord.* **20** (Suppl 12): S119–26. doi:10.1002/mds.20552. PMID 16092101.

40. "Sla, indagini nei club. Pesticidi nel mirino". http://www.corriere.it/sport/08_ ottobre_03/sla_indagine_pesticidi_fd04f986-911c-11dd-9f28-00144f02aabc. shtml. Retrieved on 2008-10-02.

41. Wicks P, Abrahams S, Masi D, Hejda-Forde S, Leigh PN & Goldstein LH (2005) The Prevalence of Depression and Anxiety in MND, Amyotrophic Lateral Sclerosis and other Motor Neuron Disorders, Volume 6, Supplement 1, p. 147

42. Rachele MG, Mascia V, Tacconi P, Dessi N, Marrosu F (April 1998). "Conjugal amyotrophic lateral sclerosis: a report on a couple from Sardinia, Italy". *Ital J Neurol Sci.* **19** (2): 97–100. doi:10.1007/BF02427565. PMID 10935845.

43. Poloni M, Micheli A, Facchetti D, Mai R, Ceriani F (April 1997). "Conjugal amyotrophic lateral sclerosis: toxic clustering or change?". *Ital J Neurol Sci.* **18** (2): 109–12. doi:10.1007/BF01999572. PMID 9239532.

44. Camu W, Cadilhac J, Billiard M. (March 1994). "Conjugal amyotrophic lateral sclerosis: a report on two couples from southern France". *Neurology (journal)* **44** (3 Pt 1): 547–8. PMID 8145930.

45. Cornblath DR, Kurland LT, Boylan KB, Morrison L, Radhakrishnan K, Montgomery M. (November 1993). "Conjugal amyotrophic lateral sclerosis: report of a young married couple". *Neurology* **43** (11): 2378–80. PMID 8232960.

46. Corcia P, Jafari-Schluep HF, Lardillier D, Mazyad H, Giraud P, Clavelou P, Pouget J, Camu W (November 2003). "A clustering of conjugal amyotrophic lateral sclerosis in southeastern France". *Neurol.* **60** (4): 553–7. PMID 12707069.

47. [2]

48. [3]

49. [4]

50. [5]

51. [6]

52. [7]

53. [8]

54. http://webmn.alsa.org/site/PageServer?pagename=MN_homepage

55. [9]

56. [10]

REFERENCES – MOTOR NEURON DISEASE

1. *motor neuron disease* at Dorland's Medical Dictionary

2. *Types of MND* at GPnotebook

3. Motor neuron degeneration in mice that express a human Cu,Zn superoxide dismutase mutation. Science, 1994. 264(5166): p. 1772-5.

4. Brooks BR (1994). "El Escorial World Federation of Neurology criteria for the diagnosis of amyotrophic lateral sclerosis. Subcommittee on Motor Neuron Diseases/Amyotrophic Lateral Sclerosis of the World Federation of Neurology Research Group on Neuromuscular Diseases and the El Escorial "Clinical limits of amyotrophic lateral sclerosis" workshop contributors". *J. Neurol. Sci.* **124 Suppl:** 96–107. PMID 7807156.

5. "El Escorial Revisited: Revised Criteria for the Diagnosis of Amyotrophic Lateral Sclerosis - Requirements for Diagnosis". http://www.wfnals.org/guidelines/1998elescorial/elescorial1998criteria.htm. Retrieved on 2007-06-06.

6. Belsh JM (2000). "ALS diagnostic criteria of El Escorial Revisited: do they meet the needs of clinicians as well as researchers?". *Amyotroph. Lateral Scler. Other Motor Neuron Disord.* **1 Suppl 1:** S57–60. doi:10.1080/14660820052415925. PMID 11464928.

7. "A Twitch of Potential". *Time.* http://www.time.com/time/pacific/magazine/article/0,13673,503060501-1186615,00.html. Retrieved on 2006-12-30.

8. Waring, S.C *et al.* (2004). "Incidence of Amyotrophic Lateral Sclerosis and of the Parkinsonism-Dementia Complex of Guam, 1950-1989". *Neuroepidemiology* **23** (4): 192–199. doi:10.1159/000078505.

9. "Flying fox linked to disease - The Boston Globe". http://www.boston.com/news/science/articles/2003/12/09/flying_fox_linked_to_disease/. Retrieved on 2007-06-06.

10. Miller G (2006). "Neurodegenerative disease. Guam's deadly stalker: on the loose worldwide?". *Science* **313** (5786): 428–31. doi:10.1126/science.313.5786.428. PMID 16873621. http://www.sciencemag.org/cgi/content/full/313/5786/428.

11. http://www.guardian.co.uk/science/2008/nov/03/lithium-motor-neurone-disease-tria

REFERENCES – MONOMELIC AMYOTROPHY

1. *monomelic_amyotrophy* at NINDS

2. MND Association

3. Overview at Washington University

4. Gourie-Devi M, Nalini A (2001). "Sympathetic skin response in monomelic amyotrophy". *Acta Neurol. Scand.* **104** (3): 162–6. doi:10.1034/j.1600-0404.2001.00016.x. PMID 11551236.

REFERENCES – LABILE AFFECT

1. Cummings J, Arciniegas D, Brooks B, Herndon R, Lauterbach E, Pioro E, Robinson R, Scharre D, Schiffer R, Weintraub D (2006). "Defining and diagnosing involuntary emotional expression disorder". *CNS Spectr* **11** (6): 1–7. PMID 16816786.

2. Brooks BR, Thisted RA, Appel SH, *et al.* (2004). "Treatment of pseudobulbar affect in ALS with dextromethorphan/quinidine: a randomized trial". *Neurology* **63** (8): 1364–70. PMID 15505150. http://www.neurology.org/cgi/pmid lookup?view=long&pmid=15505150.

3. de Seze J, Zephir H, Hautecoeur P, Mackowiak A, Cabaret M, Vermersch P (2006). "Pathologic laughing and intractable hiccups can occur early in multiple sclerosis". *Neurology* **67** (9): 1684–6. doi:10.1212/01. wnl.0000242625.75753.69. PMID 17101907.

REFERENCES – BABINSKI'S SIGN

1. *synd*/366 at Who Named It?

2. Comptes rendus de la Société de Biologie, 1896, volume 48, page 207.

3. *plantar reflex* at Dorland's Medical Dictionary

4. Harrop JS, Hanna A, Silva MT, Sharan A (2007). "Neurological manifestations of cervical spondylosis: an overview of signs, symptoms, and pathophysiology". *Neurosurgery* **60** (1 Supp1 1): S14–20. doi:10.1227/01. NEU.0000215380.71097.EC. PMID 17204875.

5. Kumar SP, Ramasubramanian D (December 2000). "The Babinski sign- -a reappraisal". *Neurol India* **48** (4): 314–8. PMID 11146592. http://www. neurologyindia.com/article.asp?issn=0028-3886;year=2000;volume=48;issue= 4;spage=314;epage=8;aulast=Kumar. Retrieved on 2009-04-13.

REFERENCES – SUPEROXIDE DISMUTASES

1. McCord JM, Fridovich I (1988). "Superoxide dismutase: the first twenty years (1968-1988)". *Free Radic. Biol. Med.* **5** (5-6): 363–9. doi:10.1016/0891-5849(88)90109-8. PMID 2855736.

2. Brewer GJ (September 1967). "Achromatic regions of tetrazolium stained starch gels: inherited electrophoretic variation". *Am. J. Hum. Genet.* **19** (5): 674–80. PMID 4292999.

3. Corpas FJ, Barroso JB, del Río LA (April 2001). "Peroxisomes as a source of reactive oxygen species and nitric oxide signal molecules in plant cells". *Trends Plant Sci.* **6** (4): 145–50. doi:10.1016/S1360-1385(01)01898-2. PMID 11286918. http://linkinghub.elsevier.com/retrieve/pii/S1360-1385(01)01898-2.

4. Corpas FJ, Fernández-Ocaña A, Carreras A, Valderrama R, Luque F, Esteban FJ, Rodríguez-Serrano M, Chaki M, Pedrajas JR, Sandalio LM, del Río LA, Barroso JB (July 2006). "The expression of different superoxide dismutase forms is cell-type dependent in olive (Olea europaea L.) leaves". *Plant Cell Physiol.* **47** (7): 984–94. doi:10.1093/pcp/pcj071. PMID 16766574.

5. Cao X, Antonyuk SV, Seetharaman SV, Whitson LJ, Taylor AB, Holloway SP, Strange RW, Doucette PA, Valentine JS, Tiwari A, Hayward LJ, Padua S, Cohlberg JA, Hasnain SS, Hart PJ (June 2008). "Structures of the G85R variant of SOD1 in familial amyotrophic lateral sclerosis". *J. Biol. Chem.* **283** (23): 16169–77. doi:10.1074/jbc.M801522200.

6. Heinrich, Peter; Georg Löffler; Petro E. Petrides (2006). *Biochemie und Pathobiochemie (Springer-Lehrbuch) (German Edition)*. Berlin: Springer. pp. 123. ISBN 3-540-32680-4.

7. Li Y, Huang TT, Carlson EJ, Melov S, Ursell PC, Olson JL, Noble LJ, Yoshimura MP, Berger C, Chan PH, Wallace DC, Epstein CJ (December 1995). "Dilated cardiomyopathy and neonatal lethality in mutant mice lacking manganese superoxide dismutase". *Nat. Genet.* **11** (4): 376–81. doi:10.1038/ng1295-376. PMID 7493016.

8. Elchuri S, Oberley TD, Qi W, Eisenstein RS, Jackson Roberts L, Van Remmen H, Epstein CJ, Huang TT (January 2005). "CuZnSOD deficiency leads to persistent and widespread oxidative damage and hepatocarcinogenesis later in life". *Oncogene* **24** (3): 367–80. doi:10.1038/sj.onc.1208207. PMID 15531919.

9. Muller FL, Song W, Liu Y, Chaudhuri A, Pieke-Dahl S, Strong R, Huang TT, Epstein CJ, Roberts LJ, Csete M, Faulkner JA, Van Remmen H (June 2006). "Absence of CuZn superoxide dismutase leads to elevated oxidative stress and acceleration of age-dependent skeletal muscle atrophy". *Free Radic. Biol. Med.* **40** (11): 1993–2004. doi:10.1016/j.freeradbiomed.2006.01.036. PMID 16716900.

10. Sentman ML, Granström M, Jakobson H, Reaume A, Basu S, Marklund SL (March 2006). "Phenotypes of mice lacking extracellular superoxide dismutase and copper- and zinc-containing superoxide dismutase". *J. Biol. Chem.* **281** (11): 6904–9. doi:10.1074/jbc.M510764200. PMID 16377630.

11. Conwit RA (December 2006). "Preventing familial ALS: a clinical trial may be feasible but is an efficacy trial warranted?". *J. Neurol. Sci.* **251** (1-2): 1–2. doi:10.1016/j.jns.2006.07.009. PMID 17070848.

12. Al-Chalabi A, Leigh PN (August 2000). "Recent advances in amyotrophic lateral sclerosis". *Curr. Opin. Neurol.* **13** (4): 397–405. doi:10.1097/00019052-200008000-00006. PMID 10970056. http://meta.wkhealth.com/pt/pt-core/template-journal/lwwgateway/media/landingpage.htm?issn=1350-7540&volume=13&issue=4&spage=397.

13. Groner Y, Elroy-Stein O, Avraham KB, Schickler M, Knobler H, Minc-Golomb D, Bar-Peled O, Yarom R, Rotshenker S (1994). "Cell damage by excess CuZnSOD and Down's syndrome". *Biomed. Pharmacother.* **48** (5-6): 231–40. doi:10.1016/0753-3322(94)90138-4. PMID 7999984.

14. Seguí J, Gironella M, Sans M, Granell S, Gil F, Gimeno M, Coronel P, Piqué JM, Panés J (September 2004). "Superoxide dismutase ameliorates TNBS-induced colitis by reducing oxidative stress, adhesion molecule expression, and leukocyte recruitment into the inflamed intestine". *J. Leukoc. Biol.* **76** (3): 537–44. doi:10.1189/jlb.0304196. PMID 15197232.

15. Campana F, Zervoudis S, Perdereau B, Gez E, Fourquet A, Badiu C, Tsakiris G, Koulaloglou S (2004). "Topical superoxide dismutase reduces post-irradiation breast cancer fibrosis". *J. Cell. Mol. Med.* **8** (1): 109–16. doi:10.1111/j.1582-4934.2004.tb00265.x. PMID 15090266.

16. Vozenin-Brotons MC, Sivan V, Gault N, Renard C, Geffrotin C, Delanian S, Lefaix JL, Martin M (January 2001). "Antifibrotic action of Cu/Zn SOD is mediated by TGF-beta1 repression and phenotypic reversion of myofibroblasts". *Free Radic. Biol. Med.* **30** (1): 30–42. doi:10.1016/S0891-5849(00)00431-7. PMID 11134893.

REFERENCES – RILUZOLE

1. Song JH, Huang CS, Nagata K, Yeh JZ, Narahashi T (01 Aug 1997). "Differential action of riluzole on tetrodotoxin-sensitive and tetrodotoxin-resistant sodium channels". *J Pharmacol Exp Ther.* **282** (2): 707–14. PMID 9262334. http://jpet.aspetjournals.org/cgi/pmidlookup?view=long&pmid=9262334.

2. Wokke J (Sep 1996). "Riluzole". *Lancet* **348** (9030): 795–9. doi:10.1016/S0140-6736(96)03181-9. PMID 8813989.

3. Azbill RD, Mu X, Springer JE (Jul 2000). "Riluzole increases high-affinity glutamate uptake in rat spinal cord synaptosomes". *Brain Res.* **871** (2): 175–80. doi:10.1016/S0006-8993(00)02430-6. PMID 10899284. http://linkinghub.elsevier.com/retrieve/pii/S0006-8993(00)02430-6.

4. Dunlop J, Beal McIlvain H, She Y, Howland DS (01 Mar 2003). "Impaired spinal cord glutamate transport capacity and reduced sensitivity to riluzole in a transgenic superoxide dismutase mutant rat model of amyotrophic lateral sclerosis". *J Neurosci.* **23** (5): 1688–96. PMID 12629173. http://www.jneurosci.org/cgi/pmidlookup?view=long&pmid=12629173.

5. Miller RG, Mitchell JD, Lyon M, Moore DH (2007). "Riluzole for amyotrophic lateral sclerosis (ALS)/motor neuron disease (MND)". *Cochrane Database Syst Rev* (1): CD001447. doi:10.1002/14651858.CD001447.pub2. PMID 17253460.

6. van Kan HJ, Groeneveld GJ, Kalmijn S, Spieksma M, van den Berg LH, Guchelaar HJ (Mar 2005). "Association between CYP1A2 activity and riluzole clearance in patients with amyotrophic lateral sclerosis". *Br J Clin Pharmacol* **59** (3): 310–3. doi:10.1111/j.1365-2125.2004.02233.x. PMID 15752377.

7. Zarate CA, Payne JL, Quiroz J, et al. (Jan 2004). "An open-label trial of riluzole in patients with treatment-resistant major depression". *Am J Psychiatry* **161** (1): 171–4. doi:10.1176/appi.ajp.161.1.171. PMID 14702270. http://ajp.psychiatryonline.org/cgi/content/full/161/1/171.

8. Coric V, Taskiran S, Pittenger C, et al. (Sep 2005). "Riluzole augmentation in treatment-resistant obsessive-compulsive disorder: an open-label trial". *Biol Psychiatry* **58** (5): 424–8. doi:10.1016/j.biopsych.2005.04.043. PMID 15993857.

9. Mathew SJ, Amiel JM, Coplan JD, Fitterling HA, Sackeim HA, Gorman JM (Dec 2005). "Open-label trial of riluzole in generalized anxiety disorder". *Am J Psychiatry* **162** (12): 2379–81. doi:10.1176/appi.ajp.162.12.2379. PMID 16330605

REFERENCES – ARIMOCLOMOL

1. Cudkowicz ME, Shefner JM, Simpson E, *et al.* (July 2008). "Arimoclomol at dosages up to 300 mg/day is well tolerated and safe in amyotrophic lateral sclerosis". *Muscle Nerve* **38** (1): 837–44. doi:10.1002/mus.21059. PMID 18551622. http://dx.doi.org/10.1002/mus.21059.

2. Traynor BJ, Bruijn L, Conwit R, *et al.* (July 2006). "Neuroprotective agents for clinical trials in ALS: a systematic assessment". *Neurology* **67** (1): 20–7. doi:10.1212/01.wnl.0000223353.34006.54. PMID 16832072. http://www. neurology.org/cgi/pmidlookup?view=long&pmid=16832072.

3. Kalmar B, Greensmith L (2009). "Activation of the heat shock response in a primary cellular model of motoneuron neurodegeneration-evidence for neuroprotective and neurotoxic effects". *Cell. Mol. Biol. Lett.* **14** (2): 319–35. doi:10.2478/s11658-009-0002-8. PMID 19183864. http://dx.doi.org/10.2478/ s11658-009-0002-8.

4. Kieran D, Kalmar B, Dick JR, Riddoch-Contreras J, Burnstock G, Greensmith L (April 2004). "Treatment with arimoclomol, a coinducer of heat shock proteins, delays disease progression in ALS mice". *Nat. Med.* **10** (4): 402–5. doi:10.1038/nm1021. PMID 15034571. http://dx.doi.org/10.1038/nm1021.

5. Kalmar B, Greensmith L, Malcangio M, McMahon SB, Csermely P, Burnstock G (December 2003). "The effect of treatment with BRX-220, a co-inducer of heat shock proteins, on sensory fibers of the rat following peripheral nerve injury". *Exp. Neurol.* **184** (2): 636–47. doi:10.1016/S0014-4886(03)00343-1. PMID 14769355. http://linkinghub.elsevier.com/retrieve/pii/S0014488603003431.

6. Rakonczay Z, Iványi B, Varga I, *et al.* (June 2002). "Nontoxic heat shock protein coinducer BRX-220 protects against acute pancreatitis in rats". *Free Radic. Biol. Med.* **32** (12): 1283–92. PMID 12057766. http://linkinghub.elsevier.com/ retrieve/pii/S089158490200833X.

7. Kalmar B, Burnstock G, Vrbová G, Urbanics R, Csermely P, Greensmith L (July 2002). "Upregulation of heat shock proteins rescues motoneurones from axotomy-induced cell death in neonatal rats". *Exp. Neurol.* **176** (1): 87–97. PMID 12093085. http://linkinghub.elsevier.com/retrieve/pii/ S0014488602979458.

8. Benn SC, Brown RH (April 2004). "Putting the heat on ALS". *Nat. Med.* **10** (4): 345–7. doi:10.1038/nm0404-345. PMID 15057226. http://dx.doi.org/10.1038/ nm0404-345.

9. Brown IR (October 2007). "Heat shock proteins and protection of the nervous system". *Ann. N. Y. Acad. Sci.* **1113**: 147–58. doi:10.1196/annals.1391.032. PMID 17656567. http://www3.interscience.wiley.com/resolve/openurl?genre=article &sid=nlm:pubmed&issn=0077-8923&date=2007&volume=1113&spage=147.

10. Kalmar B, Novoselov S, Gray A, Cheetham ME, Margulis B, Greensmith L (October 2008). "Late stage treatment with arimoclomol delays disease progression and prevents protein aggregation in the SOD1 mouse model of ALS". *J. Neurochem.* **107** (2): 339–50. doi:10.1111/j.1471-4159.2008.05595.x. PMID 18673445. http://dx.doi.org/10.1111/j.1471-4159.2008.05595.x.

11. "Phase II/III Randomized, Placebo-Controlled Trial of Arimoclomol in SOD1 Positive Familial Amyotrophic Lateral Sclerosis - Full Text View - ClinicalTrials.gov". http://clinicaltrials.gov/ct2/show/NCT00706147. Retrieved on 2009-05-18.

12. Kürthy M, Mogyorósi T, Nagy K, *et al.* (June 2002). "Effect of BRX-220 against peripheral neuropathy and insulin resistance in diabetic rat models". *Ann. N. Y. Acad. Sci.* **967**: 482–9. PMID 12079878. http://www3.interscience.wiley.com/resolve/openurl?genre=article&sid=nlm:pubmed&issn=0077-8923&date=2002&volume=967&spage=482.

13. Sebökova E, Kürthy M, Mogyorosi T, *et al.* (June 2002). "Comparison of the extrapancreatic action of BRX-220 and pioglitazone in the high-fat diet-induced insulin resistance". *Ann. N. Y. Acad. Sci.* **967**: 424–30. PMID 12079870. http://www3.interscience.wiley.com/resolve/openurl?genre=article&sid=nlm:pubmed&issn=0077-8923&date=2002&volume=967&spage=424.

REFERENCES – IPLEX

1. Williams RM, McDonald A, O'Savage M, Dunger DB (March 2008). "Mecasermin rinfabate: rhIGF-I/rhIGFBP-3 complex: iPLEX". *Expert Opin Drug Metab Toxicol* **4** (3): 311–24. doi:10.1517/17425255.4.3.311. PMID 18363546. http://www.informapharmascience.com/doi/abs/10.1517/17425255.4.3.311.

2. Kemp SF (March 2007). "Mecasermin rinfabate". *Drugs Today* **43** (3): 149–55. doi:10.1358/dot.2007.43.3.1079876. PMID 17380212. http://journals. prous.com/journals/servlet/xmlxsl/pk_journals.xml_summaryn_pr?p_JournalId=4&p_RefId=1079876.

3. Kemp SF, Thrailkill KM (April 2006). "Investigational agents for the treatment of growth hormone-insensitivity syndrome". *Expert Opin Investig Drugs* **15** (4): 409–15. doi:10.1517/13543784.15.4.409. PMID 16548790. http://www. informapharmascience.com/doi/abs/10.1517/13543784.15.4.409.

4. Jennifer Corbett Dooren (2009-03-10). "FDA Allows Use of Drug for ALS". *Wall Street Journal*. http://online.wsj.com/article/SB123672769945188703.html. Retrieved on 2009-03-11.

5. Amy Harmon (2009-05-17). "Fighting for a Last Chance at Life". *The New York Times*. http://www.nytimes.com/2009/05/17/health/policy/17untested.html. Retrieved on 2009-05-17.

6. Sorenson EJ *et al.* Subcutaneous IGF-1 is not beneficial in 2-year ALS trial. Neurology. 2008 Nov 25;71(22):1770-5

7. Jeffrey,Susan. [http://www.medscape.com/viewarticle/584247 "No Benefit of Treatment With IGF-1 in ALS"], "Medscape", 2008-11-26. Retrieved in 2008-12-06.

REFERENCES – METHYLCOBALAMIN

1. Double-blind test on the efficacy of methylcobalamin on sleep-wake rhythm disorders

2. [1]

REFERENCES – ALS ASSOCIATION

1. Mission, Vision & Values - The ALS Association

2. The ALS Association's TREAT ALS Program (Translational Research Advancing Therapy for ALS)

3. New Law Passed to Create First National ALS Registry

4. A Secretary Establishes ALS as a Presumptive Compensable Illness

5. Full List of ALS Association Chapters

6. Walk to Defeat ALS - The ALS Association

GNU FREE DOCUMENTATION LICENSE

0. PREAMBLE

The purpose of this License is to make a manual, textbook, or other functional and useful document "free" in the sense of freedom: to assure everyone the effective freedom to copy and redistribute it, with or without modifying it, either commercially or noncommercially. Secondarily, this License preserves for the author and publisher a way to get credit for their work, while not being considered responsible for modifications made by others.

This License is a kind of "copyleft", which means that derivative works of the document must themselves be free in the same sense. It complements the GNU General Public License, which is a copyleft license designed for free software.

We have designed this License in order to use it for manuals for free software, because free software needs free documentation: a free program should come with manuals providing the same freedoms that the software does. But this License is not limited to software manuals; it can be used for any textual work, regardless of subject matter or whether it is published as a printed book. We recommend this License principally for works whose purpose is instruction or reference.

1. APPLICABILITY AND DEFINITIONS

This License applies to any manual or other work, in any medium, that contains a notice placed by the copyright holder saying it can be distributed under the terms of this License. Such a notice grants a world-wide, royalty-free license, unlimited in duration, to use that work under the conditions stated herein. The "Document", herein, refers to any such manual or work. Any member of the public is a licensee, and is addressed as "you". You accept the license if you copy, modify or distribute the work in a way requiring permission under copyright law.

A "Modified Version" of the Document means any work containing the Document or a portion of it, either copied verbatim, or with modifications and/or translated into another language.

A "Secondary Section" is a named appendix or a front-matter section of the Document that deals exclusively with the relationship of the publishers or authors of the Document to the Document's overall subject (or to related matters) and contains nothing that could fall directly within that overall subject. (Thus, if the Document is in part a textbook of mathematics, a Secondary Section may not explain any mathematics.) The relationship could be a matter of historical connection with the subject or with related matters, or of legal, commercial, philosophical, ethical or political position regarding them.

The "Invariant Sections" are certain Secondary Sections whose titles are designated, as being those of Invariant Sections, in the notice that says that the Document is released under this License. If a section does not fit the above definition of Secondary then it is not allowed to be designated as Invariant. The Document may contain zero Invariant Sections. If the Document does not identify any Invariant Sections then there are none.

The "Cover Texts" are certain short passages of text that are listed, as Front-Cover Texts or Back-Cover Texts, in the notice that says that the Document is released under this License. A Front-Cover Text may be at most 5 words, and a Back-Cover Text may be at most 25 words.

A "Transparent" copy of the Document means a machine-readable copy, represented in a format whose specification is available to the general public, that is suitable for revising the document straightforwardly with generic text editors or (for images composed of pixels) generic paint programs or (for drawings) some widely available drawing editor, and that is suitable for input to text formatters or for automatic translation to a variety of formats suitable for input to text formatters. A copy made in an otherwise Transparent file format whose markup, or absence of markup, has been arranged to thwart or discourage subsequent modification by readers is not Transparent. An image format is not Transparent if used for any substantial amount of text. A copy that is not "Transparent" is called "Opaque".

Examples of suitable formats for Transparent copies include plain ASCII without markup, Texinfo input format, LaTeX input format, SGML or XML using a publicly available DTD, and standard-conforming simple HTML, PostScript or PDF designed for human modification. Examples of transparent image formats include PNG, XCF and JPG. Opaque formats include proprietary formats that can be read and edited only by proprietary word processors, SGML or XML for which the DTD and/or processing tools are not generally available, and the machine-generated HTML, PostScript or PDF produced by some word processors for output purposes only.

The "Title Page" means, for a printed book, the title page itself, plus such following pages as are needed to hold, legibly, the material this License requires to appear in the title page. For works in formats which do not have any title page as such, "Title Page" means the text near the most prominent appearance of the work's title, preceding the beginning of the body of the text.

A section "Entitled XYZ" means a named subunit of the Document whose title either is precisely XYZ or contains XYZ in parentheses following text that translates XYZ in another language. (Here XYZ stands for a specific section name mentioned below, such as "Acknowledgements", "Dedications", "Endorsements", or "History".) To "Preserve the Title" of such a section when you modify the Document means that it remains a section"Entitled XYZ" according to this definition.

The Document may include Warranty Disclaimers next to the notice which states that this License applies to the Document. These Warranty Disclaimers are considered to be included by reference in this License, but only as regards disclaiming warranties: any other implication that these Warranty Disclaimers may have is void and has no effect on the meaning of this License.

2. VERBATIM COPYING

You may copy and distribute the Document in any medium, either commercially or noncommercially, provided that this License, the copyright notices, and the license notice saying this License applies to the Document are reproduced in all copies, and that you add no other conditions whatsoever to those of this License. You may not use technical measures to obstruct or control the reading or further copying of the copies you make or distribute. However, you may accept compensation in exchange for copies. If you distribute a large enough number of copies you must also follow the conditions in section 3.

You may also lend copies, under the same conditions stated above, and you may publicly display copies.

3. COPYING IN QUANTITY

If you publish printed copies (or copies in media that commonly have printed covers) of the Document, numbering more than 100, and the Document's license notice requires Cover Texts, you must enclose the copies in covers that carry, clearly and legibly, all these Cover Texts: Front-Cover Texts on the front cover, and Back-Cover Texts on the back cover. Both covers must also clearly and legibly identify you as the publisher of these copies. The front cover must present the full title with all words of the title equally prominent and visible. You may add other material on the covers in addition. Copying with changes limited to the covers, as long as they preserve the title of the Document and satisfy these conditions, can be treated as verbatim copying in other respects.

If the required texts for either cover are too voluminous to fit legibly, you should put the first ones listed (as many as fit reasonably) on the actual cover, and continue the rest onto adjacent pages.

If you publish or distribute Opaque copies of the Document numbering more than 100, you must either include a machine-readable Transparent copy along with each Opaque copy, or state in or with each Opaque copy a computer-network location from which the general network-using public has access to download using public-standard network protocols a complete Transparent copy of the Document, free of added material. If you use the latter option, you must take reasonably prudent steps, when you begin distribution of Opaque copies in quantity, to ensure that this Transparent copy will remain thus accessible at the stated location until at least one year after the last time you distribute an Opaque copy (directly or through your agents or retailers) of that edition to the public.

It is requested, but not required, that you contact the authors of the Document well before redistributing any large number of copies, to give them a chance to provide you with an updated version of the Document.

4. MODIFICATIONS

You may copy and distribute a Modified Version of the Document under the conditions of sections 2 and 3 above, provided that you release the Modified Version under precisely this License, with the Modified Version filling the role of the Document, thus licensing distribution and modification of the Modified Version to whoever possesses a copy of it. In addition, you must do these things in the Modified Version:

A. Use in the Title Page (and on the covers, if any) a title distinct from that of the Document, and from those of previous versions (which should, if there were any, be listed in the History section of the Document). You may use the same title as a previous version if the original publisher of that version gives permission.

B. List on the Title Page, as authors, one or more persons or entities responsible for authorship of the modifications in the Modified Version, together with at least five of the principal authors of the Document (all of its principal authors, if it has fewer than five), unless they release you from this requirement.

C. State on the Title page the name of the publisher of the Modified Version, as the publisher.

D. Preserve all the copyright notices of the Document.

E. Add an appropriate copyright notice for your modifications adjacent to the other copyright notices.

F. Include, immediately after the copyright notices, a license notice giving the public permission to use the Modified Version under the terms of this License, in the form shown in the Addendum below.

G. Preserve in that license notice the full lists of Invariant Sections and required Cover Texts given in the Document's license notice.

H. Include an unaltered copy of this License.

I. Preserve the section Entitled "History", Preserve its Title, and add to it an item stating at least the title, year, new authors, and publisher of the Modified Version as given on the Title Page. If there is no section Entitled "History" in the Document, create one stating the title, year, authors, and publisher of the Document as given on its Title Page, then add an item describing the Modified Version as stated in the previous sentence.

J. Preserve the network location, if any, given in the Document for public access to a Transparent copy of the Document, and likewise the network locations given in the Document for previous versions it was based on. These may be placed in the "History" section. You may omit a network location for a work that was published at least four years before the Document itself, or if the original publisher of the version it refers to gives permission.

K. For any section entitled "Acknowledgements" or "Dedications", Preserve the Title of the section, and preserve in the section all the substance and tone of each of the contributor acknowledgements and/or dedications given therein.

L. Preserve all the Invariant Sections of the Document, unaltered in their text and in their titles. Section numbers or the equivalent are not considered part of the section titles.

M. Delete any section entitled "Endorsements". Such a section may not be included in the Modified Version.

N. Do not retitle any existing section to be entitled "Endorsements" or to conflict in title with any Invariant Section.

O. Preserve any Warranty Disclaimers.

If the Modified Version includes new front-matter sections or appendices that qualify as Secondary Sections and contain no material copied from the Document, you may at your option designate some or all of these sections as Invariant. To do this, add their titles to the list of Invariant Sections in the Modified Version's license notice. These titles must be distinct from any other section titles.

You may add a section entitled "Endorsements", provided it contains nothing but endorsements of your Modified Version by various parties—for example, statements of peer review or that the text has been approved by an organization as the authoritative definition of a standard.

You may add a passage of up to five words as a Front-Cover Text, and a passage of up to 25 words as a Back-Cover Text, to the end of the list of Cover Texts in the Modified Version. Only one passage of Front-Cover Text and one of Back-Cover Text may be added by (or through arrangements made by) any one entity. If the Document already includes a Cover Text for the same cover, previously added by you or by arrangement made by the same entity you are acting on behalf of, you may not add another; but you may replace the old one, on explicit permission from the previous publisher that added the old one.

The author(s) and publisher(s) of the Document do not by this License give permission to use their names for publicity for or to assert or imply endorsement of any Modified Version.

5. COMBINING DOCUMENTS

You may combine the Document with other documents released under this License, under the terms defined in section 4 above for modified versions, provided that you include in the combination all of the Invariant Sections of all of the original documents, unmodified, and list them all as Invariant Sections of your combined work in its license notice, and that you preserve all their Warranty Disclaimers.

The combined work need only contain one copy of this License, and multiple identical Invariant Sections may be replaced with a single copy. If there are multiple Invariant Sections with the same name but different contents, make the title of each such section unique by adding at the end of it, in parentheses, the name of the original author or publisher of that section if known, or else a unique number. Make the same adjustment to the section titles in the list of Invariant Sections in the license notice of the combined work.

In the combination, you must combine any sections entitled "History" in the various original documents, forming one section entitled "History";

likewise combine any sections entitled "Acknowledgements", and any sections entitled "Dedications". You must delete all sections entitled "Endorsements."

6. COLLECTIONS OF DOCUMENTS

You may make a collection consisting of the Document and other documents released under this License, and replace the individual copies of this License in the various documents with a single copy that is included in the collection, provided that you follow the rules of this License for verbatim copying of each of the documents in all other respects.

You may extract a single document from such a collection, and distribute it individually under this License, provided you insert a copy of this License into the extracted document, and follow this License in all other respects regarding verbatim copying of that document.

7. AGGREGATION WITH INDEPENDENT WORKS

A compilation of the Document or its derivatives with other separate and independent documents or works, in or on a volume of a storage or distribution medium, is called an "aggregate" if the copyright resulting from the compilation is not used to limit the legal rights of the compilation's users beyond what the individual works permit. When the Document is included in an aggregate, this License does not apply to the other works in the aggregate which are not themselves derivative works of the Document.

If the Cover Text requirement of section 3 is applicable to these copies of the Document, then if the Document is less than one half of the entire aggregate, the Document's Cover Texts may be placed on covers that bracket the Document within the aggregate, or the electronic equivalent of covers if the Document is in electronic form. Otherwise they must appear on printed covers that bracket the whole aggregate.

8. TRANSLATION

Translation is considered a kind of modification, so you may distribute translations of the Document under the terms of section 4. Replacing Invariant Sections with translations requires special permission from their copyright holders, but you may include translations of some or all Invariant Sections in addition to the original versions of these Invariant Sections. You may include a translation of this License, and all the license notices in the Document, and any Warranty Disclaimers, provided that you also include the original English version of this License and the original versions of those notices and disclaimers. In case of a disagreement between the translation and the original version of this License or a notice or disclaimer, the original version will prevail.

If a section in the Document is entitled "Acknowledgements", "Dedications", or "History", the requirement (section 4) to Preserve its Title (section 1) will typically require changing the actual title.

9. TERMINATION

You may not copy, modify, sublicense, or distribute the Document except as expressly provided for under this License. Any other attempt to copy, modify, sublicense or distribute the Document is void, and will automatically terminate your rights under this License. However, parties who have received copies, or rights, from you under this License will not have their licenses terminated so long as such parties remain in full compliance.

10. FUTURE REVISIONS OF THIS LICENSE

The Free Software Foundation may publish new, revised versions of the GNU Free Documentation License from time to time. Such new versions will be similar in spirit to the present version, but may differ in detail to address new problems or concerns. See http://www.gnu.org/copyleft/.

Each version of the License is given a distinguishing version number. If the Document specifies that a particular numbered version of this License "or any later version" applies to it, you have the option of following the terms and conditions either of that specified version or of any later version that has been published (not as a draft) by the Free Software Foundation. If the Document does not specify a version number of this License, you may choose any version ever published (not as a draft) by the Free Software Foundation.

INDEX